Adult Deliberate Firesetting

WILEY SERIES IN
FORENSIC CLINICAL PSYCHOLOGY

Edited by
Clive R. Hollin
School of Psychology, University of Leicester, UK

And

Mary McMurran
Institute of Mental Health, University of Nottingham, UK

For other titles in this series please visit www.wiley.com/go/fcp

Adult Deliberate Firesetting

Theory, Assessment, and Treatment

Theresa A. Gannon
Centre of Research and Education in Forensic Psychology
University of Kent, UK

Nichola Tyler
School of Psychology
Victoria University of Wellington, NZ

Caoilte Ó Ciardha
Centre of Research and Education in Forensic Psychology
University of Kent, UK

Emma Alleyne
Centre of Research and Education in Forensic Psychology
University of Kent, UK

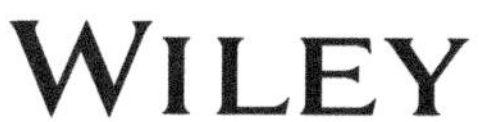

Registered Offices
John Wiley & Sons, Inc., 111 River Street, Hoboken, NJ 07030, USA
John Wiley & Sons Ltd, The Atrium, Southern Gate, Chichester, West Sussex, PO19 8SQ, UK

Editorial Office
The Atrium, Southern Gate, Chichester, West Sussex, PO19 8SQ, UK

For details of our global editorial offices, customer services, and more information about Wiley products visit us at www.wiley.com.

Wiley also publishes its books in a variety of electronic formats and by print-on-demand. Some content that appears in standard print versions of this book may not be available in other formats.

A catalogue record for this book is available from the Library of Congress

Paperback ISBN: 9781119658139; ePDF ISBN: 9781119658160; ePub ISBN: 9781119658153

Cover image: © Science photo/Shutterstock
Cover design by Wiley

Set in 9.5/12.5pt STIXTwoText by Integra Software Services Pvt. Ltd, Pondicherry, India

C103942_220322

Printed and bound by CPI Group (UK) Ltd, Croydon, CR0 4YY

For Tony Ward: Thanks for being a wonderful mentor.
Theresa A. Gannon

For my family: Thank you for encouraging me to listen and learn.
Nichola Tyler

Do Mathilde agus Maud.
Caoilte Ó Ciardha

For my parents, Noreen and Gerald Alleyne, who encouraged me to take advantage of every opportunity.
Emma Alleyne

Contents

About the Authors

Theresa A. Gannon, DPhil, CPsychol (Forensic), is a professor of forensic psychology and director of the Centre for Research and Education in Forensic Psychology (CORE-FP) at the University of Kent, UK. Theresa also works as a practitioner consultant forensic psychologist specialising in deliberate firesetting for the Forensic and Specialist Service Line, Kent and Medway Social Care and Partnership Trust, UK. Theresa has published over 150 chapters, articles, books, and other scholarly works in the areas of male- and female-perpetrated offending. She is particularly interested in the assessment and treatment of individuals who have set deliberate fires. In 2012, Theresa led the development of the first comprehensive theory of adult deliberate firesetting (named the Multi-Trajectory Theory of Adult Firesetting or M-TTAF). After leading a series of research studies examining the treatment needs of adult firesetters, Theresa developed the first standardised treatment programs for firesetters (the Firesetting Intervention Programme for Prisoners [FIPP] and Firesetting Intervention Programme for Mentally Disordered Offenders [FIP-MO]), which are now implemented in prisons and hospitals internationally. In 2016, Theresa was lead recipient of the Economic and Social Research Council's (ESRC's) Outstanding Impact in Society Award for her theoretical work and treatment provision regarding deliberate firesetting.

Theresa is lead editor of several books, including *Aggressive Offenders' Cognition: Theory, Research, and Treatment* (2007: Wiley); *Female Sexual Offenders: Theory, Assessment, and Treatment* (2010: Wiley-Blackwell); and *Sexual Offending: Cognition, Emotion, and Motivation* (2017: Wiley-Blackwell). Theresa is also co-editor of several other books. Key examples include *Firesetting and Mental Health* (2012: Royal College of Psychiatrists); *What Works in Offender Rehabilitation: An Evidence-Based Approach to Assessment and Treatment* (2013: Wiley-Blackwell); and *The Psychology of Arson: A Practical Guide to Understanding and Managing Adult Deliberate Firesetters* (2015: Routledge).

Nichola Tyler, PhD, is a lecturer in forensic psychology at Victoria University of Wellington, New Zealand. Nichola completed her PhD in forensic psychology in 2015 at the University of Kent, UK. Both her PhD and post-doctoral research focused on understanding firesetting by adults with a diagnosed mental illness. Nichola now leads the Firesetting and Forensic Mental Health Lab (FFMH Lab) at Victoria University of Wellington, where she continues to conduct research on deliberate firesetting by both youth and adults. Nichola has published over 40 journal articles, book chapters, and professional publications on the topics of deliberate firesetting, sexual offending, and rehabilitation. Nichola developed one of the first micro-theories of adult deliberate firesetting (the Firesetting Offence Chain for Mentally Disordered Offenders [FOC-MD]) and led the evaluation of the first standardised treatment programme for adults with a mental illness who have set deliberate fires (FIP-MO). On the basis of this work, she received the 2016 Kent and Medway NHS Trust Achievement in Research Award and was highly commended in the Early Career Researcher category in the 2016 Kent Innovation Awards. Alongside her academic roles, Nichola has experience of working in secure services with men and women who have set deliberate fires. She has also provided training to professionals internationally on understanding, assessing, and treating individuals with deliberate firesetting.

Caoilte Ó Ciardha, PhD, is a senior lecturer in forensic psychology at the University of Kent, UK. He completed his PhD in forensic cognitive psychology at Trinity College Dublin in 2010. His research focuses on the role and function of psychological factors in the aetiology of offending behaviours and in desistance from offending. Caoilte is particularly interested in models of offending that employ a social cognition framework. He works predominantly on the problems of sexual aggression and deliberate adult firesetting. Caoilte has published over 40 journal articles or other scholarly works on offending behaviour and holds associate editor positions at *Psychology, Crime and Law* and *Sexual Abuse*. In 2016, his research on adult firesetting was recognised as co-recipient of the ESRC's Outstanding Impact in Society Award. He is a regular contributor to television documentaries—typically in the Irish language—including *Finné: Scéal Martin Conmey*, winner of the Law Society of Ireland Justice Media Award for Human Rights/Social Justice Reporting 2019. Caoilte has received research funding from organisations, including the National Organisation for the Treatment of Abuse, the police, and UNICEF.

Emma Alleyne, PhD, is a reader in forensic psychology at the University of Kent, UK. She completed her BSc (honours) in psychology at McMaster University (Canada), followed by her MSc and PhD in forensic psychology at the University of Kent. Emma has published over 40 journal articles, book chapters, and government reports on the topics of gang-related violence, sexual offending, firesetting, and animal abuse. Her theoretical and empirical work broadly examines the social, psychological, and behavioural factors that explain various types of aggressive behaviour. Emma now leads a research programme on the aetiological factors associated with animal abuse. She has developed the first ever offence process model of animal abuse, highlighting the interactions between distal and proximal factors unique to this type of offending. Her more recent work has involved the use of innovative methods (e.g., cognitive tasks, virtual reality) to pursue research lines that investigate how offence-supportive attitudes predispose individuals to harm animals and the regulatory processes involved in triggering this type of offending behaviour. In addition to her research activities, Emma has experience working as a practitioner in secure settings delivering individual and group-based offending behaviour programmes.

Preface

When we first began examining the area of adult firesetting in the 2000s, writing a book on the topic would have been almost impossible. There was very little psychological theory or research and large gaps in our understanding of this topic. We are delighted to say that, since 2010—in particular because of the Gannon and Pina (2010) review on the topic—this picture has changed somewhat. In fact, it has changed so much that we have now been able to write a book on the topic. Our initial idea for this book stemmed from our training provision in the area of adult firesetting. We have been providing training on this topic since around 2011 and quickly realised that in order to give delegates a comprehensive overview of the topic, we had to piece together and disseminate varying sources (i.e., book chapters and journal articles). As the years have gone by, the absence of an authored book in this area has become more apparent. We sincerely hope that this book will fix this gap and promote momentum for theorists, researchers, and treatment providers who are working with adult-perpetrated firesetting. If readers take one message from this book, we hope it will be that future work in firesetting must be grounded in best practice scientific principles. This is an incredibly important field of research—a public health issue (Tyler et al., 2019a)—so it is vital that future research is well-planned and adequately powered to provide the field with the well-founded evidence and theoretical direction it requires.

Theresa A. Gannon,
Nichola Tyler,
Caoilte Ó Ciardha,
and Emma Alleyne

September 2021

Acknowledgments

We would like to acknowledge all of the individuals who have made this book possible. First of all, thank you to all of the researchers and professionals who have taken the time to research this fascinatingly complex crime. There is no doubt that this book would not have been possible without your efforts. We would also like to thank all those at Wiley-Blackwell who gave specialist advice and support on this book. In particular, thank you, Darren Lalonde, for dealing with our initial book proposal. A big thank you to everyone at Wiley-Blackwell for being so patient with us when various factors (such as a global pandemic) delayed things at our end. In particular, thanks must go to Richie Samson (project editor) and Monica Rogers (associate editor). We would also like to extend our thanks to Skyler Van Valkenburgh for helping us with the book cover and Natalie Gentry for gathering and polishing our references. Finally, we would like to thank Katie Sambrooks for helping with the final proofreading of this book and Danielle Shaw for doing the copyediting associated with this book.

1

Deliberate Firesetting

A Prevalent Yet Neglected Clinical Issue

Deliberate firesetting represents a major global public health issue (Tyler et al., 2019a). As such, criminal justice and mental health responses need to be aligned in order to be effective in reducing this type of (re)offending. The evidence base to inform prevention and intervention strategies has, until fairly recently, lacked robust, comparative designs to comprehensively capture whether individuals who set fires have unique characteristics that require tailored rehabilitation approaches. Further, aetiological theories, drawing on the limited evidence base, have typically lacked scope and explanatory power (see Hooker, 1987 or Ward et al., 2006). Likely driven by a recognition of the human cost of firesetting globally and the lack of literature outlining ways of working with this population, there has been a surge over the past decade in research outputs that rigorously and systematically addresses this gap in knowledge. With this surge have come methodological challenges. In this chapter, we review issues pertaining to definitional and measurement constraints. We also present the wider context in which firesetting literature is situated, highlighting some of the founding pillars on which recent research developments are based. The aim of this chapter is to introduce researchers and practitioners to the key concepts and disciplines that have shaped our current understanding of deliberate firesetting in adults.

Definitions, Terms, and Labels

Clear, consistently used terms and definitions enable developments in science and clinical practice alike. They also act as aide memoires to the varying motivations underpinning the aims and objectives of their use, whether it be for legal records and/or comparative research. To date, various terms have been used in the literature that refer to the deliberate and often criminal act of setting fires. *Arson*—most commonly defined as the intentional destruction of property, using fire, for unlawful purposes—is a legal term that is internationally recognised (Kolko, 2002; Williams, 2005). When used in research, *arson* typically refers to officially recorded incidents (e.g., charge, offence, conviction). As a result, research that adopts this term and definition is typically limited to known or documented incidents of fire. A further limitation is that the term *arson* does not account for people who are not convicted of arson despite having set deliberate fires (Dickens et al., 2012). Sometimes, for example, a deliberately set fire may not reach the burden of proof necessary for an arson conviction,

Adult Deliberate Firesetting: Theory, Assessment, and Treatment, First Edition. Theresa A. Gannon, Nichola Tyler, Caoilte Ó Ciardha and Emma Alleyne.

or the individual who set the fire may have escaped official detection by authorities. Clinicians often work with clients who disclose criminal behaviour not officially recorded. However, the behaviour, and its associated criminogenic factors, still warrant attention.

In the clinical context, the fifth edition of the *Diagnostic and Statistical Manual of Mental Disorders* (DSM-5; American Psychiatric Association [APA], 2013) outlines a diagnosis of *pyromania* for individuals who (1) deliberately set fire on more than one occasion; (2) experience affective and/or physiological arousal prior to the firesetting incident; (3) exhibits a fascination with fire; (4) experiences pleasure, gratification, or relief when interacting with fire and/or its consequences. This diagnosis, however, is significantly constrained by exclusion criteria. In order to be diagnosed with pyromania, the firesetting cannot have been motivated by financial gain, socio-political ideology, revenge, or the desire to cover up other criminal behaviour or improve one's living situation. The firesetting must also not have occurred in the context of psychotic symptoms, intellectual impairment, or intoxication and should not be best explained by any other diagnoses (i.e., conduct disorder, mania, antisocial personality disorder). Given these constraints, it is unsurprising that pyromania diagnoses are very rare (Gannon & Pina, 2010; Ó Ciardha et al., 2017). Consequently, researchers have had limited ability to examine any possible pyromania aetiology. In fact, given the rarity of pyromania diagnoses, the utility of such a concept for researchers or treatment professionals is at best questionable.

The term *firesetting* or *fire setting* refers to any act of deliberately setting fire. This wide-ranging umbrella term is the domain within which clinicians typically operate. That is, the term *firesetting* captures varied motivations and clinical symptomatology, as well as incidents both officially and unofficially recorded. As such, the term *firesetting* is used throughout this book except when describing research that focusses specifically on one of the subset terms described earlier. The term *fire-raising* also appears in the literature, typically used synonymously with firesetting. While it was used frequently in some older sources—notably in some influential works by Prins and colleagues (e.g., Prins, 1994)—it appears to have fallen out of favour in more recent writing. This may be due to the verb *to set* being more frequently used in general speech than *to raise* when talking about starting fires. Additionally, fire-raising has a specific legal meaning in the Scottish legal system (i.e., similar to arson) and may therefore be best avoided in favour of *firesetting* when talking about the behaviour more broadly than its legal definition(s). As with fire-raising, the term *fire-starting* occasionally appears in the literature but less frequently than firesetting. In fact, this term appears to be more frequently used in research focusing specifically on the ignition of fires rather than the wider behaviour of setting deliberate fires. Using a single term consistently—in this case, *firesetting*—helps ensure that researchers can quickly identify relevant research when searching the literature.

It is worth noting that we use person-first language in this book when referring to individuals who have set deliberate fires, who have committed other crimes, or who have a psychological disorder. This reflects a change from how many authors, including ourselves, have written about these populations in the past but brings our use of language in line with a wider de-labelling movement in research and practice relating to offending behaviour (see Willis, 2018). In clinical settings, where the primary aim is to support individuals towards desistance, the use of labels—such as "firesetter" or "offender"—only serves to reinforce stigmatising attitudes (Imhoff, 2015). If the aim is indeed desistance, then the use of these labels is not only counter-intuitive, but more important, it also violates ethical codes of practice. For example, the first principle of the British Psychological Society's Code of Ethics (2018) is respect, and within this principle individuals adhering to the code should "value the dignity and worth of all persons" (p. 5). Using labels that refer to a person's past offending behaviour reduces the person's value to that of their previously negative behaviour and signals disrespect to others (e.g., employers and residential managers). For example, a practitioner working with an individual who is routinely labelled as "firesetter" could then be biased to assume the individual is likely to reoffend. These biases could influence professional decision-making regarding resettlement and reintegration opportunities. If a psychologist is meant to strive to do no harm, labelling directly contravenes this goal (Willis, 2018). It is with these core ethical principles in mind that this book actively avoids labelling the people at the heart of the rehabilitative process in order to respect their dignity and worth.

Prevalence of Deliberate Firesetting

How we define firesetting has an impact on the consistency, and sometimes validity, of how we measure its prevalence. As a result, the manner in which fire data and statistics are recorded and reported makes it difficult to establish the true prevalence of deliberate firesetting across countries (Meacham, 2020). Looking solely at conviction rates for *arson* offences would massively underestimate the scale of the problem given the low detection and clearance rates for deliberate firesetting (see Chapter 5). Additionally, in many countries, published crime statistics routinely combine criminal damage and arson offences, making it difficult to parse firesetting prevalence from other forms of property offences. From a researcher's perspective, not all data are publicly accessible or searchable by people who cannot speak the language of the reporting country if translations are not available.

Where data are available, estimates can vary wildly depending on the recording agency and the definitions used. When we examine data from the US, for example, the FBI suggest that there are approximately 13 or 14 wilfully set fires annually for every 100,000 inhabitants (Federal Bureau of Investigation, 2015, 2018b) where an investigation has determined the fire to be deliberate. However, numbers from the US National Fire Protection Association, using a broader definition of "intentional" firesetting, suggest that the annual rate of intentional firesetting may be as high as 83 incidents per 100,000 inhabitants[1] (Campbell, 2017). It is worth noting that this higher figure may also include a proportion of firesetting incidents where the cause remained undetermined or may otherwise not have met the FBI definition.

In the UK, deliberate firesetting is operationalised within government figures as fires that have been attended by the Fire and Rescue Service and the motive recorded as deliberate. The most recent statistics available for England suggest that there were approximately 122 deliberate fires per 100,000 inhabitants annually in 2019 and 2020 (Home Office, 2021). Canadian statistics for the years spanning 2015 to 2019 suggest that rates of arson incidents are consistently between 22 and 27 per 100,000 (Statistics Canada, 2021). Data from Ireland's Central Statistics Office (2016) on the number of arson incidents recorded by police in 2015 suggest that there were 37 reported arson incidents per 100,000 inhabitants.

Data reported by Ketola and Kokki (2018) suggest that Finnish rescue services recorded approximately 20 deliberate fires per 100,000 residents.

Smith et al. (2014) used data from four Australian states to estimate the number of recorded victims of arson in Australia in 2011. Based on the figures calculated by Smith et al. (2014), we estimate that there were approximately 67 victims of arson for every 100,000 inhabitants in Australia at this time. These figures are broadly consistent with the annual rate per hundred thousand of arson offences recorded in one Australian state (Victoria) spanning 2011–2016, which ranged from 57 to 74 per 100,000 inhabitants (Crime Statistics Agency Victoria, n.d.). However, Smith et al. (2014) also estimated, based on Mayhew (2003), that there are two unreported arson victims for every case reported to the police, suggesting that the annual prevalence of arson victimisation in Australia may be as high as 200 per 100,000. Thus, it would be sensible to assume a similar under-reporting of arson in the other jurisdictions where rates are available.

We caution against comparing these figures cross-nationally because the methods of data collection vary considerably across jurisdictions. However, we consider it reasonable to estimate that the annual prevalence of deliberate firesetting serious enough to be reported to police or demand attention from fire services in the countries discussed may be in the range of 40–200 incidents per 100,000 inhabitants, when taking under-reporting into account (Mayhew, 2003; Smith et al., 2014). It remains an open question whether variability in these figures across countries reflects true cross-national differences in the rate of firesetting or is an artefact of differences in reporting and/or investigation practices between countries.

An alternative to examining rates of deliberate firesetting recorded in agency records is to use self-reported firesetting as an indicator of prevalence. To date, the most robust self-report study to ask about self-reported deliberate firesetting was the US National Epidemiologic Survey on Alcohol and Related Conditions (Blanco et al., 2010; Vaughn et al., 2010). This dataset, representative of the US population, included whether participants answered yes to the question "In your entire life, did you ever start a fire on purpose to destroy someone else's property or just to see it burn?" Using this broad—but property-focused—definition, approximately 1% of participants reported to have a lifetime prevalence of deliberate firesetting (Blanco et al., 2010; Vaughn et al., 2010).

As clinicians, one of the first questions asked is how prevalent is this offending behaviour? This helps to understand whether the behaviour requires resources invested to address it. The definitional and measurement issues presented thus far demonstrate that the research evidence needs to be interpreted with care and needs to be framed within the context of the criteria for which data are collected and recorded.

Adult Firesetting as a Neglected Topic of Research

Research examining the psychological factors underpinning firesetting behaviour and treatment for firesetting has undergone a sea change in the past decade or so. Prior to this, research on adult firesetting appeared occasionally in the literature and had relatively minimal impact. However, since the publication of a review of the state of the literature by Gannon and Pina in 2010, there have been year-on-year increases in the number of outputs on firesetting, which have impacted on the wider psychological and criminological litera-ture. Even older papers (e.g., Inciardi, 1970; Jackson et al., 1987) have seen notable increases in rates of citation in the past decade as a new generation of researchers revisits these canonical sources. It appears that sustained research from a number of research teams (especially in the UK and Australia) from 2010 onwards resulted in a critical mass for the topic. This critical mass was likely brought about by researchers and research funders rec-ognising that adult firesetting reflects a major public health and criminal justice concern with a large human and financial cost.

The neglect of adult firesetting as a research topic likely stems from an interaction of fac-tors. First, research on firesetting has historically focused on firesetting behaviour in chil-dren and adolescents. We will explore the reasons for this and the contribution of this literature to the understanding of adult firesetting. Second, it appears that there was a gen-eral belief that firesetting could be explained by either mental disorder (i.e., pyromania) or by general criminality (e.g., people setting fires to claim insurance or destroy evidence). Given that diagnoses of pyromania are exceptionally rare, there may have been a belief that firesetting behaviour was mostly addressable through general criminal offending pro-grams. Readers of this book will see that the evidence base now suggests that many indi-viduals who set fires have unique characteristics (see Chapter 2) requiring tailored risk assessments (see Chapter 4), and crucially, would benefit from interventions designed to target their distinct treatment needs (see Chapters 6 and 7).

Key Developments in the Childhood Firesetting Literature

The firesetting literature has had an asymmetrical focus on children who set fires despite evidence that only half of fires are set by children (Cassel & Bernstein, 2007). There are likely to be a number of reasons for this asymmetry, including (1) a lack of awareness of the preva-lence or seriousness of adult firesetting, (2) an assumption that firesetting was a *fire safety* and thus educational challenge, and (3) a belief that childhood firesetting may be indicative of serious and violent offending in adulthood (e.g., the "MacDonald triad"). Based on inter-views with 100 residents in a psychiatric facility, MacDonald (1963) concluded that the pres-ence of (1) enuresis (beyond 5 years of age), (2) animal cruelty, and (3) firesetting during their childhoods, taken together, was a prognostic indicator of future violence (operational-ised as "threats to kill"). The clinically appealing nature of this study for diagnostic and risk assessment purposes appears to have resulted in its wide-spread and continued application (Barrow et al., 2014). This is despite MacDonald's findings never being replicated. Instead, the evidence suggests that the presence of either animal cruelty or firesetting during child-hood is more indicative of dysfunctional and abusive childhoods (i.e., environments that normalise violent behaviour) rather than violent behaviour itself (Parfitt & Alleyne, 2020).

There has since been a shift away from focussing on the firesetting–violence link towards developing the understanding of the more proximal causes of firesetting behaviour. Root et al. (2008) explain that juvenile firesetting may be the outcome of child abuse and its result-ing affective and behavioural difficulties. The DSM-5 views firesetting behaviour as a feature of conduct disorder in children. That is, deliberately setting fires to destroy property (note animal cruelty as well) is a diagnostic criterion for conduct disorder—"a repetitive and per-sistent pattern of behaviour in which the basic rights of others ... are violated" (APA, 2013).

The child literature has also offered some insight into the dynamic risk factors associated with firesetting behaviour. For example, as a result of neglectful parenting styles (Slavkin, 2000) as well as the previously mentioned abusive household environments, children and adolescents who set fires develop impoverished and unsophisticated interpersonal social abilities. These abilities form the basis of their dysfunctional attachment styles (Räsänen et al., 1996). These relational issues have since been captured in the adult literature. Most notably, adults (in particular men) who set fires exhibit signs of loneliness with limited and/or unhelpful social support networks (Rice & Harris, 2008). Maladaptive attachment styles are associated with offending more broadly (e.g., Ross & Pfäfflin, 2007; Ward et al., 1996), and their role in reinforcing offending behaviour makes them highly suitable targets for treatment in adults.

In sum, this literature tells us that childhood firesetting points to maladaptive and dysfunctional childhood environments conducive of offending behaviour. But more important, it appears that a history of firesetting behaviour during childhood may be a risk factor for future firesetting in adulthood (Ducat et al., 2015). Therefore, the firesetting behaviour itself is indicative of a developmental psychopathology that supports the use of fire as a coping strategy and/or problem-solving method. This conceptualisation has been captured in the latest theories (see Chapter 3) and has significant implications for assessment (see Chapter 4) and treatment (see Chapters 6 and 7).

Sexual Offending Literature as a Guiding Framework

Given the paucity of the adult firesetting literature pre-2010, researchers turned to more established literatures (i.e., sexual offending) to inform the research agenda moving forward. However, although early theorising suggested a relationship between firesetting and sexual dysfunction, little available evidence substantiates this link as a major explanatory factor for adult firesetting (Ó Ciardha, 2015). Research on sexual offending has nonetheless been influential in developing knowledge relating to firesetting. This is likely the result of the longstanding recognition of sexual offending—particularly child sexual abuse—as a public health problem in need of sustained research to develop knowledge for prevention and treatment. As a result, the burgeoning field of research on deliberate adult firesetting has been able to draw on practices and concepts from the more established field of research on sexual offending.

A key influence of the field of sexual offending on firesetting research has been work by Tony Ward and various collaborators. The Multi-Trajectory Theory of Adult Firesetting (M-TTAF; Gannon et al., 2012) is an example of theorising in firesetting that draws inspiration from work, including that of Ward and Beech (2006), Ward and Hudson (1998), and Ward et al. (2006), on how to effectively develop, appraise, and knit together theories in sexual offending. Models of the offence process (micro theories) of firesetting behaviour (e.g., Barnoux et al., 2015; Tyler et al., 2014) also used methods applied by Ward et al. (1995) to the investigation of the offence process of people who sexually offend against children. Furthermore, Ward hypothesised that *implicit theories* (Ward, 2000; Ward & Keenan, 1999) and *offence scripts* (Ward & Hudson, 2000) form part of an explanatory framework for the offence-supportive belief systems of people who commit sexual offences. These concepts have been highly influential in theory development (e.g., Butler & Gannon, 2015; Ó Ciardha

& Gannon, 2012; see Chapter 3) and empirical research (e.g., Barrowcliffe et al., 2019; Butler & Gannon, 2021) on firesetting behaviour.

Changes and developments in the treatment of sexual offending over the past number of decades have also influenced current practice in the treatment of firesetting. For example, those interested in best practice with people who have sexually offended have been confronted with questions around dealing with clients who deny or minimise their offending. Similarly practice regarding treatment of sexual offending has had to navigate whether treatment ethos is most effective using a risk-based or a strengths-based approach. Building from the evidence base around what works for sexual offending has allowed contemporary intervention programmes for people who have been apprehended for firesetting (see Chapters 6 and 7) to be developed, conscious of principles of risk, need, and responsivity (Andrews & Bonta, 2010) and strength-based approaches to treatment (Good Lives Model; Ward & Stewart, 2003). These intervention programmes have been able to avoid the pitfalls faced by early sexual offending practice whereby denial and minimisation posed barriers to treatment involvement (Maruna & Mann, 2006).

Book Rationale

This chapter has provided some of the context surrounding the emergence, in the past decade and a half, of research on deliberate adult firesetting as a coherent field of enquiry. Given the relative nascence of this field, some may ask whether an entire book devoted to the assessment and treatment of adults who set fires is necessary.

At times, firesetting has been viewed as one behaviour amongst a broad repertoire of offending, whereby the individual is generally antisocial (i.e., the *generalist hypothesis*; Gannon et al., 2013). There is some research evidence to suggest that people who set fires are likely to also commit other types of offences (e.g., Soothill et al., 2004), and they are more likely to recidivate in ways other than firesetting (see Chapter 4). Based on these findings, it could be argued that firesetting does not warrant special attention. However, there is a growing body of evidence that support the *specialist hypothesis*—that some people who set fires do not commit other forms of offending—or that people with firesetting convictions may represent a distinct population within correctional settings (Gannon et al., 2013). In other words, it appears that many individuals with a history of adult firesetting have distinct psychological and psychopathological features (see Chapter 2) that require a more tailored approach to treatment. Such targeting of these likely criminogenic needs is fundamental to the effectiveness of forensic clinical practice (see Bonta & Andrews, 2017).

The fact that emerging literature suggests that people who set fires represent a population within the criminal justice and healthcare systems that experience specific needs demonstrates how our understanding of deliberate adult firesetting has changed in a short period of time. We argue that this book is timely because it allows us to synthesise the findings of a rapidly expanding field while highlighting where the gaps remain in our knowledge and where new ways of working are needed in terms of the data that public agencies and researchers gather; the manner in which researchers approach hypothesis testing around the aetiology, assessment, and treatment of people who set fires; and the ways in which practitioners work with this population.

Concluding Remarks

This book consolidates the research evidence into a practical guide to inform the assessment and treatment of adults who set fires. Evidence-based practice is the ultimate goal. However, admittedly, many elements of this book are *evidence-informed* (Bonta & Andrews, 2017) rather than evidence-based. As discussed in this chapter and further interrogated throughout this book, the research literature is yet to be saturated with clinical trials and/or quasi-experimental research designs evaluating varying methods to assess risk and reduce reoffending. Nonetheless, existing theories and research do provide sufficient steer for clinicians to make informed judgements.

Note

1 If firesetting rates were not reported per 100,000 in the sources we cite, we calculated this rate based on the reported firesetting statistic relative to the approximate population size in the relevant year. Doing so allowed us to report prevalence of firesetting in a standardised way across studies or sources.

2

Key Characteristics and Clinical Features of Individuals Who Set Deliberate Fires

Describing the characteristics of *who sets fires* will not be particularly informative unless we begin by noting two important considerations. First, there is no one personality or psychopathology that defines individuals who set fires. These individuals are heterogeneous in their characteristics, offending histories, and motives for setting fires. Second, consideration of the factors that differentiate people who engage in criminal firesetting (i.e., apprehended or non-apprehended) from people in the general population who have not engaged in criminal behaviour differs from consideration of the factors that differentiate people who have engaged in criminal firesetting from other justice-involved individuals who have not set fires. This distinction is important. If people who set fires are indistinguishable— psychologically speaking—from the general population, then practitioners have no treatment targets to address in prevention or treatment initiatives. If individuals apprehended for firesetting are indistinguishable from other justice-involved individuals, then treatments need not be tailored for firesetting. This chapter examines the key demographic, developmental, psychopathological, and psychological features of individuals who have set fires. A key aim of this chapter is to highlight (1) the key clinical features that appear to differentiate those who have set deliberate fires from the wider population and (2) the key clinical features that differentiate individuals apprehended for firesetting from other justice-involved individuals.

When considering the characteristics of any offending population, it is worth considering why we are interested in these characteristics. First, establishing what sets our focal population apart from the rest of the population may provide indirect evidence of the causal chains that have led to the offending behaviour. The observation of differences between groups provides a starting point for hypothesising about the causal relationships between background or psychological factors and offending behaviours like firesetting. Second, examining group differences in characteristics helps us to determine which factors are statistically related to increased risk of offending or re-offending and thus improves decisions about the prioritisation of individuals for treatment as well as public protection decisions about release and supervision. A third reason why we are interested in the characteristics of offending populations is to determine which factors may be targets for treatment.

A key consideration when examining and presenting information on the characteristics of adults who set fires is the quality of evidence available. The most useful evidence for the characteristics of this population would come from high-quality sources, ideally cohort studies, representative large sample studies, well-powered studies with matched comparison groups, or meta-analyses. Unfortunately, these types of sources are rare in the study of adult firesetting due to the relative recency of sustained research on the topic.

Characteristics of Adults Who Set Fires

Sociodemographic Findings

Men appear more likely to engage in deliberate firesetting than females. Examination of a nationally representative US sample including participants self-reporting lifetime firesetting (including juvenile firesetting) suggested that for every woman reporting deliberate firesetting, there were almost five men (the National Epidemiologic Survey on Alcohol and Related Conditions [NESARC] dataset; Blanco et al., 2010; Hoertel et al., 2011; Vaughn et al., 2010). A study of all individuals convicted of arson in Sweden over a 12-year period indicated that approximately four men were convicted of arson for every woman (Anwar et al., 2011). The gender difference was slightly larger in a study of all individuals convicted of arson in a 9-year period in a single Australian state, with over six men convicted for every woman (Ducat et al., 2017). Dickens and Sugarman (2012) suggested that women may be more likely to be diverted from the criminal justice system or referred to psychiatric services. Some psychiatric samples appear to evidence this latter point. For example, Enayati et al. (2008) reported three men for every woman in their study of all individuals convicted of arson and sent for psychiatric assessment over a four-year period in Sweden. While men appear to set deliberate fires at a higher rate than women, women appear to account for a higher proportion of those convicted of firesetting than they do of people convicted of other offences (Ducat et al., 2013a). To date, research appears only to have examined firesetting and gender using a male–female dichotomy.

There is little clear evidence that ethnicity meaningfully intersects with whether people set fires. Using nationally representative self-reported US data, lifetime firesetting was reported less frequently by Black, Hispanic, and Asian participants than by non-Hispanic white participants (Blanco et al., 2010). However, this dataset (the NESARC study; see also Hoertel et al., 2011; Vaughn et al., 2010) is one of few sources of prevalence statistics using nationally representative data. Another US representative study of adolescents also indicated that self-reported firesetting was more common among white participants than participants of other ethnicities (Chen et al., 2003). However, the dearth of comparable non-US literature presents a challenge in generalising any ethnicity difference in self-reported firesetting prevalence to other jurisdictions. Dickens and Sugarman (2012) concluded that the ethnicity of individuals who set fires in existing clinical studies is broadly comparable to the population from which they are drawn. For example, Gannon (2010) suggested that women who set fires were characterised by white ethnicity. However, this was consistent with individuals apprehended for other offences in the small sample studies she relied on and likely matched the general population in those jurisdictions.

The population of apprehended adults who set fires appear to be more likely than non–justice-involved individuals to experience greater socioeconomic disadvantage and have lower educational attainment, as well as lower rates of skilled employment (for a review, see Gannon & Pina, 2010). Based on a small number of studies that compared people who set fires to other apprehended individuals, individuals with a history of firesetting appear to have lower attainment in terms of education (Räsänen et al., 1995) and employment (Ducat et al., 2013a; Räsänen et al., 1995). However, when we look at the NESARC data on self-reported firesetting in the US population, it appears that individuals who had set fires were not characterised by sociodemographic differences compared with the wider community (Blanco et al., 2010; Vaughn et al., 2010). Split by gender (Hoertel et al., 2011), these same data suggest that men who set fires had *higher* levels of education on average than those who had not set fires. Across three UK studies, Barrowcliffe and Gannon (2015, 2016; Gannon & Barrowcliffe, 2012) found no clear evidence of sociodemographic differences between individuals reporting firesetting for which they had not been apprehended and people who did not report firesetting.

The current literature is very limited in scope in terms of its examination of the sociodemographic characteristics of adults who set fires. However, based on what is currently available, adults who set fires do not appear to differ profoundly from the rest of the population apart from a clear predominance of men, a potentially higher prevalence among white individuals, and lower socio-economic status and educational attainment. Further research is needed that compares appropriate samples of adults who set fires to other justice involved individuals on basic demographic variables.

Developmental Context

Early factors—including genetic, biological, neurodevelopmental, and experiential factors—have been variously hypothesised as distal causal factors in adult firesetting. The results of Swedish population research (Frisell et al., 2011) suggests that there are genetic or early developmental influences on the commission of arson among those aged 15 years or older. To our knowledge, little additional research has been carried out to further determine the specific mechanisms through which genes may act on the psychological processes underpinning firesetting behaviour.

Research on neurobiological factors in firesetting has not advanced considerably since a review by Gannon and Pina (2010). Among the most promising research on the neurobiology of firesetting was research by Virkkunen and colleagues that implicated a role for certain neurotransmitters in distinguishing between people apprehended for arson and other offending groups as well as in predicting recidivism among people apprehended for arson (Virkkunen et al., 1987, 1989). Specifically examining the evidence of neurobiological characteristics for individuals who have set fires and have a mental disorder, Tyler and Gannon (2012) concluded that the literature is reliant on case studies or very small samples, limiting the conclusions that can be drawn.

Low IQ has been historically associated with adult firesetting. Nanayakkara et al. (2015) summarised the available evidence, concluding that while high rates of intellectual disability appeared to characterise some samples of individuals who have set fires, low IQ does not necessarily distinguish individuals who have set fires from other justice-involved individuals. A meta-analysis of four studies (predominantly adult samples) found that rates of intellectual disability among individuals with a history of firesetting appear to be less than

5% (Sambrooks et al., 2021; see also Collins et al., 2021 for a systematic review that also reports autism prevalence).

Gannon and Pina (2010) drew together literature suggesting that the developmental backgrounds of individuals who set fires are characterised by adversity. Specifically, they identified research (e.g., Bradford, 1982; McCarty & McMahon, 2005) implicating larger families, parental neglect, and sexual and physical abuse as factors differentiating young people and adults who set fires from other justice-involved individuals or from the wider population. In the decade since their review, very little research has examined whether the developmental experiences of people who set fires are markedly different to other groups. One exception is a paper by Ducat et al. (2013a), which compared a sample of men and women with convictions for firesetting offences with case files of randomly selected convicted individuals without firesetting histories. Both groups were characterised by childhood adversity but did not appear to differ meaningfully from one another. It is worth noting that there may be within-group variability in childhood adversity for people who have set fires, evidenced by the finding that individuals who set multiple fires may be characterised by greater physical and sexual abuse in childhood (Bell et al., 2018).

Taken together, the early lives of people who set deliberate fires in adulthood appear to be characterised by biological and experiential factors that differentiate them from the population of people who do not encounter the criminal justice system. There is also tentative evidence that genetic and neurobiological factors may differentiate people who set fires compared with those involved in other forms of criminality. There is less evidence of clear differences between the developmental experiences of people who set fires compared with other justice-involved individuals. Overall, the general picture of the developmental context of firesetting behaviour is of a literature that needs considerable updating with large robust studies.

Mental Disorder and Psychopathology

Firesetting behaviour has been consistently linked with mental ill health. The Multi-Trajectory Theory of Adult Firesetting (M-TTAF; Gannon et al., 2012) conceptualises mental health as a moderator of the link between causal factors and firesetting. In other words, mental ill health may exacerbate underlying risk factors to make firesetting more likely (see also McEwan & Ducat, 2016). This reflects a departure from some earlier views that presented a more direct, causal link between mental disorder and certain firesetting behaviour (e.g., Prins, 1994). Broadly speaking, the empirical research has focused on specific areas of mental disorder or psychopathology when it comes to a possible role in firesetting—pyromania, personality disorder, disorders involving psychosis, substance misuse, affective or mood disorders, and anxiety disorders.

Pyromania. Pyromania is perhaps the most obvious mental disorder to consider as linked to firesetting behaviour (and likely more causally than as a moderator). It is defined by multiple occasions of deliberate firesetting combined with tension or arousal prior to setting the fire and pleasure, gratification, or relief following setting the fire according to the fifth edition of the *Diagnostic and Statistical Manual of Mental Disorders* (DSM-5; American Psychiatric Association, 2013). Furthermore, there must be evidence of interest, curiosity, or attraction towards fire. However, there is little evidence of diagnostic utility of the concept of pyromania due to the number of exclusionary criteria included in the DSM (see Ó Ciardha et al., 2017). In fact, among populations of individuals apprehended for firesetting, a diagnosis of pyromania is extremely rare (e.g., Lindberg et al., 2005; Sambrooks et al., 2021). A key reason for the rarity of pyromania diagnoses is that DSM-5 exclusion criteria stipulate that firesetting should not be better accounted for by conduct disorder, mania, or antisocial personality disorder.

Personality disorders. The research examining personality disorders and firesetting has commonly implicated antisocial personality disorder as well as borderline personality disorder. Meta-analytic findings suggest that approximately one third of individuals apprehended for firesetting may have a personality disorder (Sambrooks et al., 2021). In summarising this literature, Nanayakkara et al. (2015; see also Tyler & Gannon, 2012) concluded that while antisocial personality disorder appears to characterise individuals who set fires (e.g., Lindberg et al., 2005; Repo et al., 1997; Vaughn et al., 2010)—and in particular those who use fire within a varied pattern of offending—borderline personality disorder and traits typically distinguish people apprehended for firesetting from other apprehended individuals (e.g., Ducat et al., 2013b; Duggan & Shine, 2001; Ó Ciardha et al., 2015a). Synthesising results across prison, secure mental health settings, and research on the wider population, personality disorder appears to be particularly characteristic of women who set fires when compared with men who have set fires and with other women (Alleyne et al., 2016; Hoertel et al., 2011; Nanayakkara et al., 2020a; Wyatt et al., 2019).

Psychosis. Psychosis and psychotic disorders (e.g., schizophrenia) have also been reported as comorbid with or otherwise linked with firesetting behaviour (Dickens & Sugarman, 2012; Nanayakkara et al., 2015; Sambrooks et al., 2021; Tyler & Gannon, 2012). Firesetting may even act as a marker for the subsequent onset of schizophrenia or schizoaffective disorder in some cases (Thomson et al., 2017). One of the most robust studies examining psychosis and a possible link with firesetting was carried out by Anwar and colleagues (2011) using a case-control design and a large sample of Swedish participants, including all individuals convicted of arson in a 13-year period. Both men and women with convictions for arson were more likely than population controls to have diagnoses of schizophrenia or other psychoses. Another well-powered study replicated the finding that there are differences between firesetting and community samples in terms of psychotic disorders, this time with a mixed-gender Australian sample (Ducat et al., 2013b). However, psychotic disorders did not differentiate individuals apprehended for firesetting from other justice-involved individuals in their sample, except when they looked specifically at schizophrenia, which was over-represented among individuals who had set fires. Using the NESARC US data, rates of self-reported diagnoses of psychotic disorders did not appear to be more prevalent among people with a history of firesetting compared with people without (Blanco et al., 2010; Vaughn et al., 2010). However, when split by gender (Hoertel et al., 2011), the same data indicated that women with a firesetting history were more likely to report psychotic disorder than women without. Psychosis and psychotic disorders also appear to be more strongly characteristic of women apprehended for arson compared with men apprehended for arson and women without firesetting histories (e.g., Anwar et al., 2011; Enayati et al., 2008).

Substance dependence. Some of the early conclusions of an association between substance dependence and adult firesetting (see, e.g., Gannon & Pina, 2010) were based on a literature limited by small sample sizes or lack of comparison groups (Grant & Kim, 2007; Lindberg et al., 2005; Ritchie & Huff, 1999). A number of more recent robust studies appear to support these initial conclusions (Alleyne et al., 2016; Blanco et al., 2010; Ducat et al., 2013b; Hoertel et al., 2011; Ó Ciardha et al., 2015a; Sambrooks et al., 2021; Vaughn et al., 2010). Sambrooks et al. (2021) reported meta-analytic findings suggesting that two thirds of individuals with a history of firesetting in their samples had diagnoses for substance-related issues. Nationally representative US data suggested that drug and alcohol use disorders were characteristic of men and women with a lifetime history of firesetting compared with those without (Blanco et al., 2010; Hoertel et al., 2011; Vaughn et al., 2010). Comparing a large sample of individuals convicted of arson offences with offending and community individuals, Ducat et al. (2013b) found that frequency of substance misuse diagnoses were higher for people who had set fires than either of the two other groups. Breaking down the same firesetting sample by gender, Ducat et al. (2017) reported that women who had set fires were more likely than men to have a psychiatric diagnosis of substance misuse. Two related studies looking at the psychopathology of men and women with and without firesetting histories imprisoned in the UK examined the presence as well as the prominence of drug dependence in these individuals (the male participants in these studies overlapped; Alleyne et al., 2016; Ó Ciardha et al., 2015a). Male participants who had set fires showed greater presence and prominence of drug dependence than imprisoned men who had not set fires (Ó Ciardha et al., 2015a). Women who had set fires were broadly similar to men who had set fires in terms of the presence of drug dependence but appeared slightly higher in terms of the prominence of the syndrome (Alleyne et al., 2016). Imprisoned women without a history of firesetting, however, had the highest rates of drug dependence overall. Higher rates of alcohol dependence appeared to differentiate men and women who set fires from those who did not across these two studies (Alleyne et al., 2016; Ó Ciardha et al., 2015a).

Affective and anxiety disorders. Affective and/or anxiety disorders appear to co-occur regularly with firesetting behaviour (Dickens & Sugarman, 2012). Examination of the US NESARC dataset suggested that bipolar and anxiety disorders were more prevalent among people sampled in the community who set fires compared with people with no history of firesetting (Blanco et al., 2010). Compared with a community sample, individuals with convictions for firesetting were found by Ducat et al. (2013b) to have a greater frequency of bipolar, depressive, and anxiety disorder diagnoses. When compared with other individuals receiving a criminal charge, depressive and anxiety disorder diagnoses were still more frequent among people who had set fires, but bipolar diagnoses did not differentiate between the groups. The absolute number of individuals with bipolar disorder diagnoses in any group was relatively small. When Ducat and colleagues (2017) examined the same data to compare women and men who had set fires, they found again that the small number of individuals with bipolar disorder diagnoses did not differentiate men from women, nor did anxiety disorders. However, diagnoses of depressive disorders were significantly more frequent among women in their data. Using a self-report measure of psychopathology, Ó Ciardha et al. (2015a) found that imprisoned men with a history of firesetting reported more traits associated with anxiety, dysthymia, and major depression but not bipolar disorder compared with other men in the criminal justice system. In a related study, it was the presence of bipolar disorder and major depression that appeared to differentiate imprisoned women with a history of firesetting from men who had set fires or other imprisoned women (Alleyne et al., 2016).

There are caveats to consider when synthesising the available evidence of psychopathology and firesetting. There are very few tightly controlled large sample studies contributing to the knowledge base in this area; exceptions include Anwar et al. (2011), Ducat et al. (2013b), and studies using the NESARC data (Blanco et al., 2010; Hoertel et al., 2011; Vaughn et al., 2010). As a result, much of what we know about the psychopathology of this population is based on small opportunity samples or higher quality studies whose findings may be specific to the jurisdictions sampled. These findings may also be affected by the broader confound of whether people are apprehended or imprisoned for their firesetting. Provisionally, however, it is possible to conclude that the available evidence points to firesetting as a behaviour that is frequently comorbid with mental disorders and mental ill health and that this comorbidity is more pronounced than in other justice-involved individuals. Women who set fires appear to hold higher rates of psychopathology relative to men.

Psychological Traits

The findings we have presented so far have focused on developmental trajectories or the presence or absence of diagnosable mental health issues in men and women who set fires. In this section, we explore the psychological traits that have been associated with those who engage in firesetting behaviour. We have used the M-TTAF (Gannon et al., 2012) to arrange these psychological traits into four categories reflecting what Gannon and colleagues consider *psychological* vulnerabilities—inappropriate fire interest or scripts, offence-supportive attitudes, self- or emotion-regulation issues, and communication problems. We also examine self-esteem, which is conceptualised as a moderator within the M-TTAF in that self-esteem may buffer the individual against the impact of their underlying vulnerabilities on firesetting behaviour (Gannon et al., 2012). It is important to acknowledge that these psychological traits may not be independent of the psychopathological and developmental factors already examined. For example, fire interest is *the* defining feature of pyromania, and aspects of poor self-regulation may typify people with intellectual disability. This is therefore a different lens with which to view the characteristics of this population, which reflects a different level of analysis to the examination of disorders or development (for a discussion of the examination of offending phenomena at different levels of analysis, see Ward, 2014).

Fire interest and fire scripts. Fire interest refers, predictably, to whether individuals experience a marked or inappropriate interest in fire, fire paraphernalia, or other facets surrounding firesetting behaviour (e.g., interest in the emergency service response to fires). It is a core feature of pyromania but alone is not sufficient for a diagnosis of pyromania (see Ó Ciardha et al., 2017). Unsurprisingly, fire interest is consistently associated with firesetting status. Factor analytic research by Ó Ciardha et al. (2015b) suggested that it may be useful to distinguish between an interest in mundane firesetting (e.g., an ordinary fire in a grate) and more serious firesetting (e.g., a hotel fire). They found that this serious firesetting factor distinguished imprisoned men who had set fires from those who had not (for similar findings in a well-matched subset of these data, see Gannon et al., 2013). Similarly, Alleyne et al. (2016) reported data suggesting that imprisoned women who had set fires had greater serious fire interest than imprisoned women who had not set fires. Two studies by Barrowcliffe and Gannon (2015, 2016) did not distinguish fire interest according to its severity yet reported greater fire interest among un-apprehended individuals admitting firesetting compared with the general population. Tyler et al. (2015) demonstrated greater prevalence of expressed fire interest—as recorded in clinical notes—for individuals in a secure mental health setting who had set fires than those who had not.

Recently, Gannon et al. (in preparation), developed a comprehensive self-report tool to examine fire-related interests and attitudes. For a more detailed description of the measure, see Chapter 6. Factor analysis of responses from a large community sample, including individuals admitting deliberate firesetting, allowed the authors to parse fire-related attitudes more finely than earlier studies (e.g., Ó Ciardha et al., 2015b). All eight factors extracted from the measure differentiated between people admitting a history of firesetting and those who did not. Factors labelled as *identification with fire, fire interest, pathological fire interest, coping using fire*, and *fascination with fire paraphernalia* appear to reflect facets of fire interest. In a second study, Gannon et al.'s (in preparation) findings suggest that it is the coping using fire and identification with fire facets of fire interest that best differentiate between imprisoned men with and without convictions for firesetting.

Gannon et al. (2012) hypothesised that individuals who set deliberate fires may have developed cognitive scripts that facilitate firesetting (this theory was further developed by Butler & Gannon, 2015). Very little research has empirically tested the scripts of people who have set fires. Using a relatively small sample, Butler and Gannon (2021) found evidence of greater fire-related scripts and expertise among imprisoned men with current or previous firesetting offences compared with community and imprisoned individuals. Interestingly, fire-service personnel were indistinguishable from people who had set fires using Butler and Gannon's measures of scripts and expertise, and both groups scored similarly on serious fire interest. Gannon et al.'s (in preparation) examination of the structure and correlates of a new measure of fire-related interests and attitudes provides additional evidence regarding firesetting scripts through the identification of coherent factors approximating two of Butler and Gannon (2015) hypothesised scripts: fire is a powerful messenger, and fire is soothing.

Offence-supportive attitudes. Gannon et al. (2012) hypothesised that adults who set deliberate fires would hold attitudes supportive of general offending and/or specific attitudes that would support criminal firesetting. Ó Ciardha and Gannon (2012) expanded on this hypothesis by proposing that people who set fires may have belief systems in the form of *implicit theories* (see Ward, 2000) that allow them to interact with their social words and process social information in an offence-supportive manner. We know of only one published study that has directly tested these hypotheses. Barrowcliffe et al. (2019) found only partial support for the specific hypotheses of Ó Ciardha and Gannon (2012) with a small sample of un-apprehended individuals (majority female) who had set fires. The findings of Gannon et al. (in preparation) also appear to support the suggestion by Ó Ciardha and

Gannon (2012) that the belief that fire is a powerful tool may be characteristic of people who set fires as well as beliefs around how fascinating or exciting fire is.

Self and emotional regulation. The self- or emotion-regulation factors implicated in adult deliberate firesetting by the authors of the M-TTAF (Gannon et al., 2012) include issues with anger, poor coping or emotional expression, poor problem solving, and impulsivity. As mentioned, these factors may reflect clinical features of certain developmental disabilities or psychopathological disorders. However, they are not simply hypothesised as features of broader disorders but also as vulnerability factors in people who set fires in the absence of diagnosed mental ill health. Much of the older research on which these hypotheses were drawn relied on small samples or samples without comparison groups. Few studies have directly explored whether these factors distinguish groups of individuals who have set fires from other justice-involved individuals or the wider community. Gannon et al. (2013) compared imprisoned men with and without firesetting offences on a number of variables, including anger. They found that those with firesetting histories appeared to be characterised by more anger-related cognition (e.g., rumination and hostility) and physiological arousal to anger and had more experiences of anger as a response to perceived provocation. Findings by Alleyne et al. (2016) suggested that apprehended women who had set fires reported being *more* able to regulate their anger relative to other imprisoned women, although the effect size for this difference was small. Comparing a small sample of women and men who had set fires, Nanayakkara et al. (2020a) reported greater impulsivity and affect dysregulation among the female sample. Impulsivity also differentiated women who had set fires from other women admitted to a secure treatment setting (Long et al., 2015). Taking a different approach, Dalhuisen et al. (2017) examined the evidence for different subgroups of firesetting individuals. They concluded that some clusters of these individuals were characterised by self- or emotion-regulation factors such as coping problems or problems with impulsivity. Finally, Gannon et al. (in preparation) found that self and emotional regulation among people who set fires may be characterised by a reliance on fire as a method of coping or as a means to send a powerful message to others. These factors differentiated apprehended individuals with a history of firesetting from both apprehended and community controls.

Communication problems. Within the M-TTAF (Gannon et al., 2012), communication problems that are thought to act as vulnerabilities for firesetting include social skills issues, emotional loneliness, and low assertiveness. As with other factors, early research implicated these as characteristic of people who set fires (see Gannon & Pina, 2010), but a few more recent studies have demonstrated whether they are uniquely characteristic of this population. Gannon et al. (2013) did not find group differences between imprisoned men who set fires compared with those who did not on either assertiveness or loneliness using self-report measures. Alleyne et al. (2016) found that these social competence measures of loneliness and assertiveness did not differentiate imprisoned women who had set fires from other imprisoned women or from the men who had set fires. In one of few relatively recent studies that examined the social skills of people who have set fires, Hagenauw et al. (2015) reported lower social skills among the small sample of firesetting individuals in their comparison of mixed-gender individuals in a psychiatric institution. In a study that compared men apprehended for arson with men apprehended for violent offences and who were treated in an outpatient treatment centre, Wilpert et al. (2017) found that those apprehended for arson were more socially isolated.

Self-esteem. Self-esteem is conceptualised within the M-TTAF (Gannon et al., 2012; see Chapter 3) as a moderating factor, with intact or high self-esteem potentially protecting individuals against the deleterious effects of other psychological vulnerabilities that would otherwise place them at risk of offending. In this model, low self-esteem may exacerbate these risk factors. The best evidence of this relationship would demonstrate that self-esteem interacts with other risk factors preceding firesetting offending. However, evidence that individuals who engage in firesetting have lower self-esteem than comparison groups would provide partial support for this hypothesis. Two studies have reported significantly lower self-esteem among imprisoned men with a history of firesetting compared with imprisoned individuals (Duggan & Shine, 2001; Gannon et al., 2013). Analyses by Alleyne et al. (2016) has also suggested that while imprisoned women who set deliberate fires had lower self-esteem than men who set fires, they did not differ significantly from other imprisoned women (though see also Stewart, 1993). The possibility that gender may itself impact on a moderating role of self-esteem was suggested by Ducat et al. (2017).

Relative to research on the psychopathological characteristics of individuals who set fires, research on psychological characteristics is less well-developed. There appears to have been a resurgence in this area of investigation following publication of the M-TTAF (Gannon et al., 2012). However, the lack of routinely available national or regional data (c.f., Anwar et al., 2011; Ducat et al., 2013b) on these psychological characteristics impedes the development of robust large-scale examination of these constructs and their potential role in firesetting. Despite this, the cumulative evidence is strongest in implicating fire interest (or facets of fire interest), self- and emotion-regulation problems, and low self-esteem as characteristics of men who have set fires relative to other justice-involved men. Fire interest also appears to consistently differentiate between people who have set deliberate fires and the wider population and between women who set fires and other imprisoned women. Other findings relating to women are less clear and require further research using robust designs. There is growing evidence to consider fire interest as multi-faceted and that firesetting may be underpinned by firesetting-supportive schemas and scripts, but these need further investigation.

Characteristics of Subgroups of Adults Who Set Fires

The research on characteristics of adults who set fires is dominated by studies that imply a certain homogeneity in the life events and the psychological or psychopathological vulnerabilities of these individuals. In other words, research often pits a group of individuals who have set deliberate fires against a group of individuals who have not. This approach risks oversimplifying a nuanced and complex phenomenon. Both theory (e.g., Gannon et al., 2012) and research on motives or typologies in firesetting (e.g., Lewis & Yarnell, 1951) paint the picture of a much more heterogeneous population following varied offence pathways (see also Barnoux et al., 2015; Tyler & Gannon, 2017). Therefore, it is important to think beyond the very general characteristics of people who set fires and instead consider finer-grained distinctions within this population. We have already examined the interaction of gender and firesetting status in the earlier sections. However, researchers have also investigated the characteristics of specific subsets of individuals who set fires, including those who engage in repeated firesetting or high-consequence firesetting, as well as those whose firesetting may belong to specific typologies or trajectories.

The rates of recorded firesetting recidivism are relatively low (Ducat et al., 2015; Rice & Harris, 1996; Thomson et al., 2018). Sambrooks et al. (2021) meta analysed studies looking at reoffending by untreated adults or children with a history of firesetting. They again found relatively low rates of reoffending (8%–10%) when considering reoffending as convictions (or arrests or charges in one study) for "arson". Using a broader definition of firesetting, however, the reoffending rate was higher (20%). Doley et al. (2011) summarised a limited literature on the characteristics of individuals who set repeated fires. They also identified a number of promising target areas for future research on recidivism in this population. The following decade has seen publication of some robust examinations of repeat firesetting, though there remains a lot of potential for further research in this area. Synthesising this literature, the strongest evidence of characteristics of repeat firesetting includes having fire interest (Dickens et al., 2009; Tyler et al., 2015), more past firesetting incidents (Ducat et al., 2015; Rice & Harris, 1996), young age at first firesetting (Dickens et al., 2009; Rice & Harris, 1996), being criminally versatile (Dickens et al., 2009; Ducat et al., 2015), personality disorder (Dickens et al., 2009; Thomson et al., 2018; Wyatt et al., 2019), intellectual disability (Bell et al., 2018), and childhood adversity (Bell et al., 2018; Dickens et al., 2009).

Dickens and colleagues (2009) highlighted the need to parse the dangerousness of firesetting from recidivism. They reported that few of their variables were able to predict the dangerousness of fires and those that did related to the firesetting behaviour itself rather than individual characteristics. However, building on this research Nanayakkara et al. (2020b) examined the characteristics of individuals who engaged in what they termed *high-consequence* firesetting (i.e., the setting of fires that resulted in fatality or high financial costs). They reported that high-consequence firesetting could be arranged into five types based on the clustering together of demographic, situational, and crime behaviour variables recorded in coroner files. Here, individuals whose firesetting appeared object-focused (e.g., vandalism) were typically younger, had less violence in their offending histories, and had higher rates of repeat firesetting compared with individuals whose firesetting was person-focused who had less repeat firesetting or violence in their pasts but greater symptoms of major mental illness. The nature of the data (i.e., coroners reports) with which Nanayakkara et al. (2020b) developed their typology somewhat limits what can be said about the psychological characteristics of the different groupings of individuals who set fires. However, in interpreting their typology, Nanayakkara and colleagues (2020b) argue that they provide at least partial evidence of four of five hypothetical pathways to adult firesetting proposed within the M-TTAF (Gannon et al., 2012).

Dalhuisen et al. (2017), set out explicitly to assess the trajectories of the M-TTAF using all individuals referred to a single clinic in the Netherlands over a period of over 60 years for pretrial assessment following a suspected firesetting offence. They reported that their participants appeared to cluster into five groupings. Dalhuisen et al. (2017) interpreted their findings as partially supporting the hypothesised M-TTAF trajectories. Perhaps more important for the focus of the current chapter, their findings appear to evidence considerable variability within samples of individuals who have set fires in terms of developmental (history of abuse), psychopathological (psychosis), and psychological (empathy, impulsivity, coping, and social skills) characteristics.

Limitations of the Literature and the Current Review

In summarising the literature, we have attempted to give greater weight to high-quality empirical sources as well as high-quality reviews synthesising the existing literature. Despite these aims, we have also relied in places on less robust studies, especially where those studies are more recent and have not been incorporated into past reviews.

A limitation of the adult firesetting literature to date has been the lack of comparison groups or the use of only one comparison group. As a result, it is not always possible to examine what differentiates individuals who have set fires from the wider community *and* from other justice-involved individuals. Additionally, the literature on adult firesetting has often focused on individuals who have a mental disorder *and* a history of firesetting. Given the theoretical and empirical links between psychopathology and firesetting, this focus is unsurprising. However, the sampling of individuals with a mental disorder or those without also likely reflects a pragmatic decision in terms of the population to which researchers have had access. As a result, studies of institutionalised individuals have often focused on just one type of institutional setting, either prison (e.g., Ó Ciardha et al., 2015a) or secure mental health (e.g., Wyatt et al., 2019). We have attempted to bring together the results of these studies in reviewing the available literature in this chapter and are most confident in results that appear consistent across settings.

Most psychological research on the characteristics or clinical features of individuals who set fires has been conducted in so-called WEIRD countries (i.e., Western, educated, industrialised, rich and democratic), particularly majority Anglophone as well as countries in the north of Europe. Research has focused less on a global picture of this phenomenon. Additionally, research conducted in WEIRD countries has not typically disaggregated findings to examine the generalisability of findings to ethnic minorities or indigenous populations within those countries. One exception to this trend was a recent study by Ellis-Smith et al. (2019), which examined differences in some offence characteristics (and criminal justice system outcomes) between Aboriginal and non-Aboriginal Australians who had set fires. Gannon et al. (2012) highlighted how cross-cultural differences in the use of fire and of education in its use may need to be accounted for in models of deliberate firesetting. This cross-cultural perspective remains lacking from much of the research summarised in this chapter.

Conclusions, Ways of Working, and Future Directions

Our review of the literature on the characteristics of individuals who have set deliberate fires as adults demonstrates a field that has expanded considerably in the past decade. There are clearly still gaps in our knowledge, and there remains a need for large representative studies and replication of older findings. However, the cumulative evidence appears to confirm that individuals who set fires reflect a population that—when considered in aggregate—have characteristics that set them apart from the general population across early developmental, psychopathological, and psychological domains. When compared with other justice-involved individuals, people who set fires appear to be broadly similar in terms of their sociodemographic and early developmental characteristics but may have specific vulnerabilities, risk factors, or treatment needs relating to their psychological and psychopathological characteristics.

We are encouraged by a growing move beyond examining the characteristics of homogenised groups of individuals who set fires towards examining the characteristics of subgroups of firesetting individuals. Given that the expansion of the literature that we note in this chapter, we believe that there is increasing scope to take a meta-analytic approach to synthesising knowledge on the characteristics of people who set fires. We strongly encourage practitioners and people working with populations of people who have set fires to routinely embed measures (e.g., Gannon et al., in preparation) of the psychological characteristics most clearly linked with firesetting behaviour in their assessment procedures. Doing so will help provide the foundation for future work on theory, assessment, and treatment of this population.

3

Theories of Deliberate Firesetting

Refreshing the M-TTAF

Developing theory to explain why individuals set deliberate fires is critical for understanding how best to reduce this behaviour. Deliberate firesetting is a fascinatingly complex criminal behaviour; yet relative to other criminal behaviours (e.g., violence, sexual offending), it has received little theoretical attention. In this chapter, we begin by presenting readers with the key factors associated with effective psychological theory. Then, using these criteria, we present and appraise available typological and theoretical explanations of firesetting, including a refreshed and updated version of the Multi-Trajectory Theory of Adult Firesetting (M-TTAF) (Gannon et al., 2012). Finally, we highlight key aetiological gaps that exist in this area and present ways for clinicians to work with the current theoretical literature available to them.

Effective Psychological Theory

Effective psychological theory is critical for the assessment and treatment of firesetting behaviour. Ward and colleagues (Ward & Hudson, 1998; Ward et al., 2006) were the first researchers to highlight that theories in the offending behaviour realm differ regarding level of theoretical focus. They argued that theories tend to take one of three foci: single-factor, multi-factor, or micro-process theories. *Single-factor* theories tend to exclusively focus on one factor or mechanism and its relationship to offending. *Multi-factor* theories unify various single-factor theories into a comprehensive explanation of offending behaviour. *Micro-process* theories focus on the proximal factors involved in how an offence unfolded and tend to be based on narrative self-report accounts. Ward and colleagues also highlighted several virtues that characterise sound psychological theory in the form of *empirical adequacy* (i.e., is the theory underpinned by adequate research evidence?), *unification* (i.e., does the theory synthesise previously isolated theory or research evidence?), *depth* (i.e., does the theory describe detailed processes or mechanisms?), *coherence* (i.e., does the theory provide a clear and coherent account of variables and mechanisms), and *fertility* (i.e., is the theory of value for clinical assessment or intervention purposes; see Hooker, 1987 or Schindler, 2018). In the following sections, we describe and evaluate available typological and theoretical explanations of firesetting, including a refreshed and updated version of the M-TTAF (Gannon et al., 2012) according to the criteria associated with effective psychological theory.

Typological Explanations of Firesetting

Typological explanations of firesetting are not generally regarded as theories but instead as valuable foundations for theory development (Gannon & Pina, 2010; Ward & Carter, 2019). Because of this, we will not evaluate typologies according to the criteria associated with effective psychological theory. Instead, we will describe and evaluate them more generally in order to provide context regarding theoretical explanations of firesetting. Readers interested in typological classification of firesetting more generally should consult Tyler and Gannon (2021).

Typologies generally subdivide individuals who have set fires into groups or subtypes in accordance with perceived motivations or offence characteristics (e.g., Barker, 1994; Bradford, 1982; Icove & Estepp, 1987; Inciardi, 1970; Levin, 1976; Lewis & Yarnell, 1951; Prins, 1994; Rix, 1994; Scott, 1974). These can range from very simple dichotomous typologies to more complex typologies that consist of multiple categories. For example, Scott (1974) stated that firesetting could be categorised simply as being either *motivated* or *motiveless*. Icove and Estepp (1987), on the other hand, described six categories of motive underpinning firesetting: *vandalism, excitement, revenge, profit, crime concealment*, and *undetermined*. The problem with typological approaches to firesetting, however, is that they do not tend to capture the complexity of firesetting motives since motivators are not typically excusive and often overlap or co-occur (Gannon & Pina, 2010; Tyler & Gannon, 2020). A further issue is that the methods employed in developing firesetting typologies lack standardisation. Consequently, typologies of firesetting are difficult to compare meaningfully and do not adequately account for the complexity of firesetting motives as seen in clinical practice. However, these typologies have been useful in drawing attention to the immense differences in motivators underpinning firesetting (e.g., revenge, vandalism, cry for help, profit, self-harm, excitement, crime concealment).

A further type of classificatory system used in the firesetting literature relates to criminal profiling. Here, professionals use crime scene data and data associated with perpetration characteristics to draw key conclusions about the profile of the individual who has set the fire (Canter & Fritzon, 1998; Douglas et al., 1992, 2006, 2013a; Kocsis & Cooksey, 2002). For example, using evidence from the crime scene such as accelerant use and the presence of intricate incendiary devices, the Federal Bureau of Investigation's Crime Classification Manual (Douglas et al., 1992, 2006, 2013a) describes firesetting as being either organised (i.e., crime scene evidence implies a precise and planned approach to firesetting) or disorganised (i.e., crime scene evidence implies that materials and ignition sources and accelerants were used simply due to their availability). Within this structure, various subtypes of individuals who set fires are then proposed according to key factors such as motivators and fire features. Such typologies are useful for informing investigatory processes; however, they are less useful for informing assessment and treatment of firesetting clinically.

An important development in typological approaches to firesetting are typologies that have been generated as a result of statistical analyses (Green et al., 2014; Harris & Rice, 1996; Nanayakkara et al., 2020a, 2020b). For example, Harris and Rice (1996) identified four subtypes of firesetting based on a cluster analysis of key variables collected from the inpatient files of 243 adults at a high-security psychiatric hospital in Canada. These subtypes were named *psychotics* (e.g., cluster variables highlighted delusional motivators and schizophrenia diagnoses), *unassertives* (e.g., cluster variables highlighted low levels of assertiveness and anger or revenge motivators), *multi-firesetters* (e.g., cluster variables highlighted multiple firesetting, aggression and poor developmental experiences), and *criminals* (e.g., cluster variables highlighted extensive criminal histories and a personality disorder). A strength of this approach is that numerous factors can be objectively grouped according to data patterns. However, typologies based on statistical analyses are unable to outline how the factors included in each subtype relate to each other, limiting their use in guiding assessment and treatment approaches with individuals who have set fires.

Single-Factor Theories

There are four key single-factor theories that have been proposed to explain firesetting: *psychoanalytical, biological, social learning, and script theory*. Psychoanalytical theory represents one of the earliest attempts to explain firesetting (see Freud, 1929/2000, 1932). From a psychoanalytic perspective, firesetting is believed to be caused by fixated oral/urethral psychosexual drives such that firesetting is hypothesised to be a phallic symbol that signifies sexual urges and enuresis an attempt to extinguish firesetting within dreams (Barnett & Spitzer, 1994; Gaynor & Hatcher, 1987; Kaufman et al., 1961; Vreeland & Levin, 1980). The psychoanalytical account of firesetting has been surprisingly influential in modern professional and lay rhetoric around firesetting (see Ó Ciardha, 2015c or Horsley, 2020). This may well be due to the clear and coherent account of the psychosexual factors accountable for firesetting proffered by the theory (i.e., theoretical coherence). However, sexual desires have been established in very few cases (see Barnett & Spitzer, 1994), and the key principles underlying the theory have not been adequately validated (i.e., poor empirical adequacy). Other key problems with the theory include poor explanatory depth, unification, and fertility. For example, psychoanalytical theory fails to account for key factors implicated in firesetting such as developmental experiences and has not led to intervention or treatments that reduce firesetting behaviour. Thus, psychoanalytical theory requires substantial research and clinical evidence to become a more convincing theory of firesetting.

Biological theory represents a more recent explanatory approach that has focused on impulsive or repetitive firesetting and the link with neurobiological impairments (Roy et al., 1986; Virkkunen et al., 1987, 1989). For example, Virkkunen et al. (1987) found that individuals who had set fires were characterised by decreased 5-hydroxyindoleacetic acid and 3-methoxy-4-hydroxyphenylglycol concentrations relative to approximately matched offender and non-offender comparisons. Virkkunen et al. (1989) observed that individuals who reoffended in a 3-year period ($\pm$ 18 months) were more likely to have 5-hydroxyindoleacetic acid irregularities relative to individuals who had previously set a fire but not yet reoffended. Taken together, these studies suggest that neurotransmitter deficits may be one important factor to consider when explaining repeated firesetting. A key strength of the biological approach—relative to psychoanalysis—is that it is supported by empirical evidence. It also unifies the previously isolated theory regarding neurobiological impairments with the concept of firesetting. A key problem with biological theory, however, is the lack of explanatory depth regarding exactly how neurotransmitter deficits translate into firesetting behaviour. Despite this issue, however, biological theory holds some clear potential clinical fertility since serotoninergic drugs could be used to manage 5-hydroxyindoleacetic acid irregularities.

Social learning theory explains firesetting as culminating via social learning experiences that may occur through observing or being taught by others and experiencing particular rewards or penalties (Bandura, 1976; Macht & Mack, 1968; Vreeland & Levin, 1980). For example, some professionals (e.g., Vreeland & Levin, 1980) have noted that firesetting itself holds properties that are instantly reinforcing in the form of sensory stimulation. Other positively reinforcing factors associated with fire might come from the reactions of others (e.g., praise from antisocial peers for setting a large fire or media attention that makes an individual feel powerful). Social learning theory might explain why individuals who set fires appear to originate from families or within environments where fire use is prevalent (Barnoux et al., 2015; Rice & Harris, 1991; Wolford, 1972). Social learning theory appears best suited to explaining firesetting that occurs as a result of fire interest. However, it is also able to account for firesetting that occurs in relation to anger- or revenge-based motivations. To illustrate, self-regulation is hypothesised to develop as a result of environmental reinforcement contingencies. Thus, negative developmental experiences and poor role models are likely to result in the development of key characteristics linked with revenge firesetting in the form of assertiveness and problem-solving deficits and aggression (see Gannon et al., 2012 or Butler & Gannon, 2015). Social learning theory has received some empirical support regarding the links between developmental experiences with fire and later fire misuse (see Barnoux et al., 2015). These links are also relatively clearly unified and explicated (coherence) as well as being explained with some depth. Regarding clinical fertility, social learning theory represents an appealing avenue of explanation that may be used by practitioners with their clients to understand how fire-supportive interests are developed and maintained (i.e., via conditioning principles).

Script theory (Butler & Gannon, 2015; Gannon et al., 2012) represents what is arguably the most recent single-factor explanation of firesetting behaviour. Gannon et al. (2012) first introduced the concept of a firesetting script when they published the M-TTAF described later in this chapter. They argued that individuals learn how fire should be used and in what contexts via the development of a cognitive script that initially forms during childhood (i.e., a "fire script"). Gannon et al. (2012) proposed that two key inappropriate fire scripts might explain why fire is chosen as a criminal tool amongst so many other potential tools or weapons. Interestingly, these scripts were hypothesised to form as a result of social learning theory (e.g., formative experiences of fire use). One of these was named the *fire-coping script*. For individuals who developed this script, it was hypothesised that fire becomes viewed as a powerful messenger to cope with a variety of problems since it attracts attention rapidly, destroys property permanently, and promotes rapid environmental change. The second script was named the *aggression-fire fusion script*. This refers to the formation of an indirect-aggression script (i.e., in which indirect aggression becomes a preferred method of gaining revenge or warning others) that incorporates fire as the key messenger. Presumably, fire becomes a naturally fitting key messenger due to its ability to instantaneously instil fear in others.

In 2015, Butler and Gannon elaborated the concept of firesetting script theory and proposed two additional firesetting scripts based on research evidence and their own clinical experience: *fire is a powerful messenger*, and *fire is the best way to destroy evidence*. The former script encapsulates the aggression-fire fusion script proposed by Gannon et al. (2012) but includes an additional dimension in the form of fire having been learnt to be a powerful messenger of *distress* (e.g., to elicit attention or cry for help). The latter script refers to an inappropriate script regarding the use of fire that has evolved through criminal behaviour engagement. Here, fire has come to be a preferred method of destroying evidence via criminal experience and knowledge around the destructive nature of fire. Butler and Gannon argue that this script plays a critical role in explaining how it is that individuals repeatedly misuse fire to cover up their crimes in the seeming absence of any excessive fire interest. Thus, in terms of clinical fertility, script theory is useful and appealing in the sense that it provides a clear target for interventions in cases of repeated fire use in which fire interest appears absence. Script theory has also gained a small amount of empirical support in the area of firesetting (Butler, 2018; Butler & Gannon, 2021) and holds relatively good theoretical coherence and unification through outlining the links between social learning theory and the development of scripts in the explanation of firesetting. Explanatory depth is also relatively good since Butler and Gannon (2015) provide considerable detail regarding how such scripts are likely to become formed as a result of key formative and adulthood experiences.

Micro-process Theories

Micro-process theories—sometimes referred to as offence chain theories—represent a relatively recent academic development in firesetting. These theories are generated directly from participants' descriptions of the key factors leading up to their firesetting using the qualitative method of grounded theory (Strauss & Corbin, 1998). The resultant theory provides a descriptive pictorial model of the cognition, affect, events, and contextual factors preceding, surrounding, and following a firesetting incident. Once the model has been constructed, participants are typically examined to see how they flow through the model representing the offence process and common pathways to firesetting are identified and described.

There are two key micro-process theories that have been developed to explain deliberate firesetting: the Firesetting Offence Chain for Mentally Disordered Offenders (FOC-MD; Tyler et al., 2014) and the Descriptive Model of the Offence Chain for Imprisoned Adult Male Firesetters (DMAF; Barnoux et al., 2015). Tyler et al.'s FOC-MD was developed using the offence descriptions of 23 mixed-sex individuals who had set a deliberate fire and were resident in a UK secure psychiatric hospital. Once the model had been constructed, Tyler et al. (2014) were able to identify three key patterns of firesetting that did not appear to be influenced by participant gender. These three patterns or pathways to firesetting were distinguishable on four key factors: (1) the development of fire-related risk factors such as a strong affective response to fire or interest in fire during childhood, (2) timing of mental health issue commencement, (3) the amount of fire planning utilised, and (4) whether or not the participant had stayed to watch the fire set. Individuals labelled as following the "fire interest-child mental health" pathway were characterised by the development of fire-related risk factors in childhood, longstanding mental health issues, explicit planning of their firesetting, and staying to watch the fire. Individuals identified under the "no fire interest-adult mental health" pathway, on the other hand, were notable through the absence of fire-related risk factors in childhood and adult onset of mental health issues. These individuals appeared to suddenly experience mental health issues immediately preceding their firesetting and did not generally explicitly plan or stay to watch the firesetting. Finally, individuals labelled under the "fire interest-adult mental health" pathway were characterised by the presence of fire-related risk factors and the commencement of mental health issues in adulthood. These individuals performed some lower level planning of their firesetting and only stayed to watch the fire if their circumstances allowed this.

Barnoux et al. (2015) developed the DMAF using the offence accounts of 38 male UK prisoners who had either been convicted for a firesetting offence or had set a deliberate fire in prison. After detailing the factors leading up to and around the time of each firesetting offence, Barnoux et al. (2015) were able to identify two key firesetting pathways: *approach* or *avoidance*. Individuals characterised by the approach pathway tended to have experienced difficult childhoods characterised by abuse, early incidents of fire or firesetting, and displayed antisocial behaviour and traits such as offending in childhood or adulthood and aggression. These individuals tended to approach their offence *aggressively*, planning their offence, which was typically motivated by instrumental gain or feelings of anger (e.g., revenge, protest) and often intended to endanger life. The men following this pathway towards firesetting tended to experience positive affect in relation to their firesetting and the harm caused. Individuals characterised by the avoidant pathway were also found to be characterised by a difficult childhood. However, unlike the approach individuals, they tended not to have engaged in early antisocial behaviour or had engaged to a lesser extent and were less likely to have developed fire interests and vulnerabilities (e.g., normalisation of fire) or to have been involved with fire during childhood. These individuals appeared to be characterised by passive traits (e.g., low levels of assertiveness) and were found to live largely pro-social lives prior to their firesetting. However, these individuals did report having experienced some significant and stressful life events such as death of a loved one prior to their firesetting. Individuals who followed this pathway did not appear to want to intentionally harm others through their firesetting. They tended to indirectly approach the firesetting, often "finding" themselves in a situation that led to firesetting aimed at solving a criminal problem, exerting power, or protesting over a situation they perceived as being insurmountable.

A key strength of both micro-process theories regards their ability to highlight key factors associated with firesetting. Both are based on data provided by individuals who have experience of firesetting and who are perhaps the best people to describe the intricacies of the firesetting offence process (i.e., evidence of empirical adequacy and depth). Furthermore, the FOC-MD has received additional pathway validation (Tyler & Gannon, 2017). Nevertheless, these theories are yet to attract external empirical support. Both theories unify previously isolated factors in relation to firesetting (e.g., aggressiveness and intent to endanger life in the DMAF) showing evidence of theoretical unification. However, the theoretical coherence of these theories is perhaps a little weaker given the large number of pictorial model categories that require considerable interpretation on the part of the reader. Nevertheless, the clinical fertility of the theories is considerable since both highlight the sequence of events leading to firesetting and provide clinicians with prototypical subtypes or pathways that group individuals according to motivational themes and key characteristics. Consequently, such theories may be useful for clinicians who are tasked with the role of treatment plan formulation for subtypes of individuals who have set fires.

Multi-factorial Theories

Prior to the development of the M-TTAF (Gannon et al., 2012), there were two longstanding multi-factor theories available to explain firesetting: Functional Analysis Theory (FAT; Jackson, 1994; Jackson et al., 1987) and Dynamic Behaviour Theory (DBT; Fineman, 1980, 1995). FAT was the earliest attempt to explain firesetting using multiple factors. Jackson and colleagues (1987) used clinical functional analysis to propose that firesetting onset and maintenance were the result of the interaction of antecedents (i.e., previous circumstances) and behavioural consequences (i.e., reinforcement contingencies) accompanying fire use. In brief, five key factors are proposed to underlie firesetting in the FAT (Figure 3.1): (1) *psychosocial disadvantage* (e.g., poor caregiver experiences and the accompanying psychological effects of this), (2) *life dissatisfaction and self-loathing* (e.g., depression or poor self-esteem resulting from psychosocial disadvantage), (3) *social ineffectiveness* (e.g., poor conflict resolution skills or societal rejection), (4) *factors that define an individual's fire experiences* (e.g., previous direct or vicarious fire experiences), and (5) *triggers* (e.g., emotional experiences or contexts). The FAT presents reinforcement contingencies as being key for both facilitating and maintaining firesetting. To illustrate, Jackson et al. (1987) hypothesise that fire offers socially ineffective children both power and influence over peers as well as increased attention from distracted or neglectful caregivers which positively reinforces fire use or fire interest. Thus, the combination of an increase in personal effectiveness and positive sensory stimulation is hypothesised to further increase fire interest and the associated chances of fire being used inappropriately. Jackson et al. (1987) also highlighted a key role for negative reinforcement principles in the maintenance of firesetting. They argued that firesetting often produces punitive responses in the form of punishment and intense supervision, which may serve to further establish personal inadequacies already experienced by the individual. Consequently, the problems that resulted in fire being misused to begin with become further exacerbated. Jackson (1994) argues that firesetting, from a functional analysis perspective, resolves problems or difficult issues that the individual feels are impossible to solve using alternative methods.

The FAT has been used widely by clinical professionals internationally. This is likely due to the fact that the FAT provides a clear and relatively coherent account of the variables and mechanisms involved in firesetting and its maintenance (i.e., the theory has good *coherence*) and combines conditioning theory with early knowledge regarding firesetting (i.e., the theory exhibits *unification*). Because of this, the FAT is able to provide clinicians with clear direction regarding the formulation of firesetting behaviour as well as the key targets to treat (e.g., social skills, personal effectiveness) in order to reduce firesetting (i.e., good clinical *fertility*). Some of the core tenets underlying the FAT have received empirical support (e.g., individuals who have set deliberate fires experience negative affect preceding firesetting; Barnoux et al., 2015; Murphy & Clare, 1996; Tyler et al., 2014), suggesting that the FAT holds *empirical adequacy*. As research has progressed, however, it has become clear that social competence is not

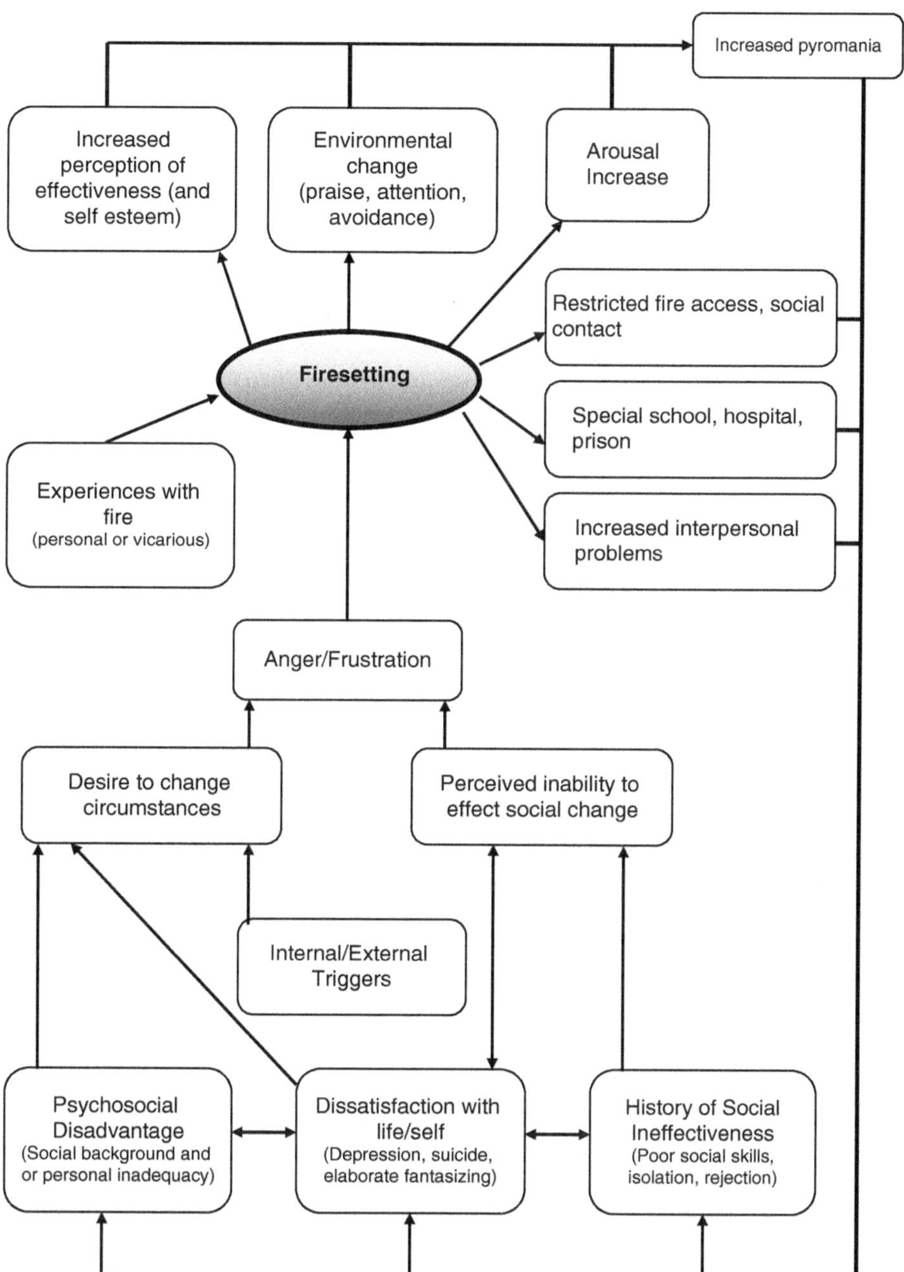

Figure 3.1   Jackson et al.'s functional formulation of recidivist arson (adapted from Jackson et al., 1987).

the primary deficit associated with firesetting behaviour (see Gannon et al., 2013), and the key factors of mental health and gender are given little consideration in the FAT (suggesting some lack of depth). Furthermore, the FAT does not explain how individuals with predominantly non-firesetting histories, who may not exhibit any fire interest, choose to misuse fire.

Similar to the FAT, DBT (Fineman, 1980, 1995) views firesetting as stemming from historical psychosocial influences that shape and direct firesetting via social learning. Fineman draws upon dynamic behavioural principles in relation to firesetting (see Cook et al., 1989; Gaynor, 1991) to propose that firesetting can be explained by the following formula:

Firesetting $= G1 + G2 + E$

in which $[E = C + CF + D1 + D2 + D3 + F1 + F2 + F3 + Rex + Rin]$

This equation explains firesetting as resulting from (G1) historical factors encouraging antisocial behaviour (e.g., social disadvantage, social effectiveness), (G2) preceding and present environmental reinforcement contingencies supporting firesetting (e.g., childhood fire experiences, fire interest), and (E) instantaneously reinforcing environmental contingencies that support firesetting (e.g., sensory stimulation). Fineman (1995) then goes on to specify that the instantly reinforcing contingencies can be further understood through exploring (C) impulsivity triggers (e.g., rejection); (CF) crime scene information about the firesetting goal; (D1, D2, and D3) cognitions before, at the time of, and after the firesetting; and (F1, F2, and F3) affective experiences before, at the time of, and after the firesetting. Reinforcers of firesetting are referred to by Fineman as R, and these may be external (Rex; e.g., evading the law) or internal (Rin; e.g., sensory stimulation). Fineman suggests that practitioners examine all of the factors encompassed by this formula in order to fully understand and formulate a specific case of firesetting.

Similar to the FAT, DBT provides a relatively clear and coherent account of the variables and mechanisms involved in firesetting and its maintenance (i.e., good *coherence*). Furthermore, many of the theory's underlying assumptions have been empirically supported illustrating a good level of *empirical adequacy* (e.g., individuals who set fires often report social disadvantage; Barnoux et al., 2015; Gannon & Pina, 2010). The theory has also successfully unified conditioning principles with firesetting knowledge (e.g., cognitive and affective reinforcers), illustrating theoretical *unification*. Similar to the FAT, DBT provides clinicians with clear direction regarding the formulation of firesetting behaviour as well as the key targets to treat (e.g., social effectiveness) in order to reduce firesetting (i.e., good clinical *fertility*). However, this theory is perhaps not as intuitively appealing for clinicians to use and like the FAT it assumes that all firesetting stems from poor developmental experiences and provides little emphasis on factors such as mental health or gender (i.e., lack of explanatory depth).

The M-TTAF (Gannon et al., 2012) was developed using the concept of theory knitting (Kalmar & Sternberg, 1988) and is the most recent multi-factor attempt to explain firesetting. The M-TTAF uses theory knitting to bring together the strongest parts of the FAT (Jackson et al., 1987; i.e., learning and reinforcement principles) and DBT (Fineman, 1980, 1995; i.e., a focus on cognition) with the firesetting research literature to explain firesetting facilitation and maintenance or desistance. The overarching M-TTAF integrates developmental, biological, social, cultural, and psychological factors to explain firesetting via two explanatory "tiers." Tier 1 is the overarching theoretical framework of the M-TTAF, and Tier 2 documents a selection of hypothesised firesetting "subtypes" that are predicted to exhibit specific characteristics from within Tier 1. Tier 1 represents the overarching aetiological framework of the M-TTAF and is presented in Figure 3.2. Within Tier 1, firesetting is conceptualised as stemming from complex interactions between an individual's developmental context, psychological vulnerabilities, proximal factors and triggers, moderators, and critical risk factors. Developmental factors incorporate aspects such as caregiver

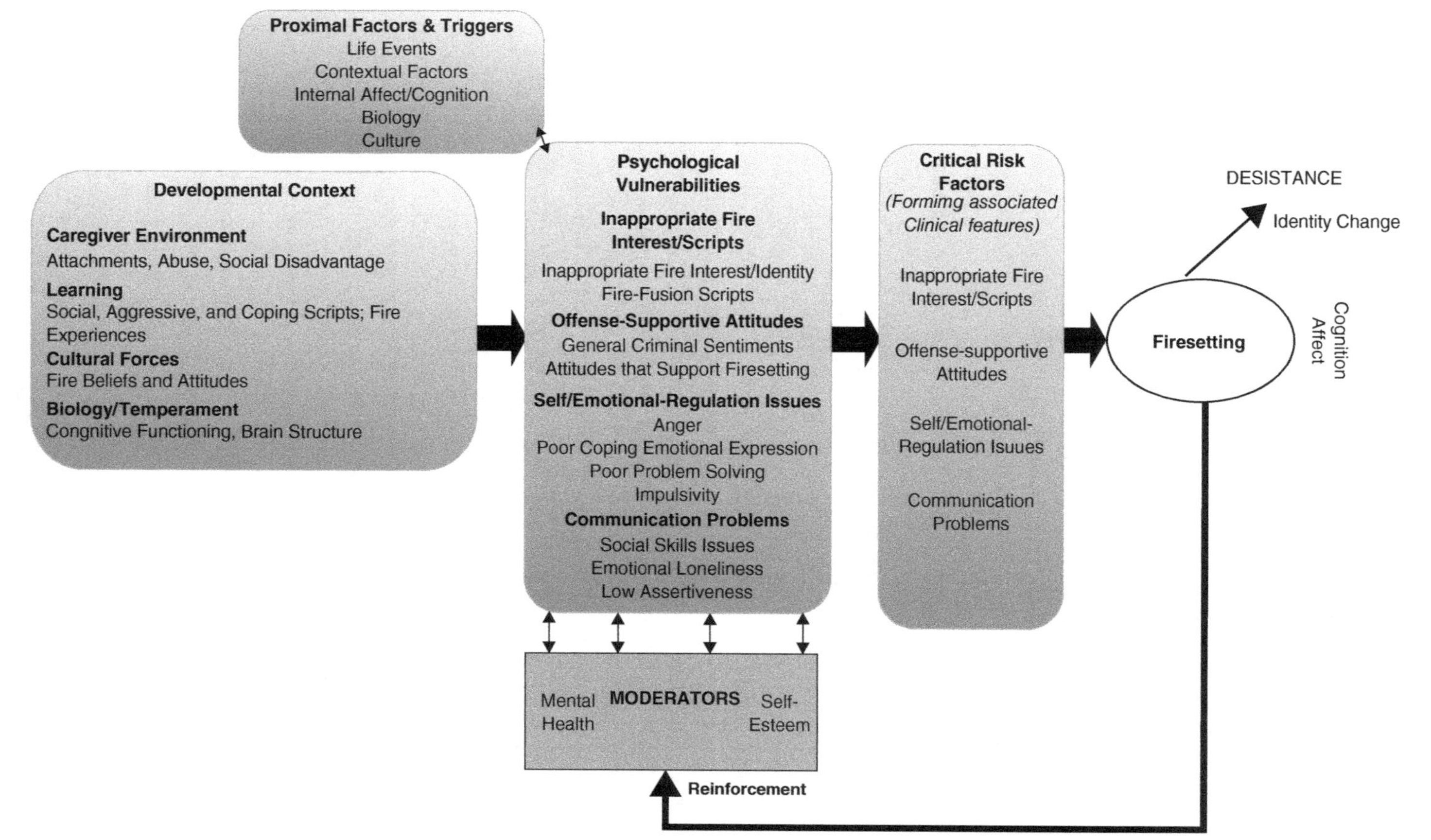

Figure 3.2 The original M-TTAF: Tier 1.

environment, learning, cultural forces, and biological or temperamental factors related to the developing child. To illustrate, a child who experiences neglectful or distracted caregivers (caregiver environment) and who exhibits poor communication and coping styles may learn early in their development that lighting fires is an excellent way of gaining attention (learning). The child's choice to use fire as a tool for communication with others might be incidental. However, it may also be influenced by cultural factors. In the Western world, for example, fire is generally regarded as "dangerous," and children are shielded from fire use. Consequently, fire gains attention from others rapidly, particularly if the fire is unexpected and potentially threatening. Some biological or temperamental factors (e.g., low IQ, impulsivity) may further facilitate the child's willingness to use fire as a method of communication. However, protective factors are also likely to shape the individual's response to negative developmental factors (e.g., high IQ, communication and self-regulation skills).

The child's developmental context results in their entering adulthood holding a unique combination of psychological vulnerabilities: *inappropriate fire interest or scripts, offence-supportive attitudes, self/emotional regulation issues,* and *communication issues.* The vulnerability of holding an inappropriate fire interest refers to a marked and inappropriate interest in fire and fire use (e.g., deliberately setting up opportunities to see fires). An inappropriate fire script—which may exist with or without inappropriate fire interest—refers to a fire-coping script or fire-aggression fusion script in which fire use becomes either a preferred mechanism for coping or a powerful indirect messenger of aggression, respectively. Offence-supportive attitudes refer to attitudes supporting offending generally (e.g., a general entitlement to offend) or that more specifically support deliberate firesetting (e.g., a belief that fire is controllable). Empathy or theory of mind issues are also important here since offence-supportive cognitions can signify issues in these areas. Theory of mind, in particular, refers to putting oneself in another's shoes (Baron-Cohen & Wheelwright, 2004) and is a factor of empathy likely to be absent when offence-supportive attitudes are present. Self/emotional-regulation issues refer to problems regulating emotional states (e.g., impulsivity, anger) as well as problematic coping styles (e.g., avoidant coping). Communication issues refer to problems with social skills, assertiveness, and the appropriate development and maintenance of both intimate and non-intimate relationships.

So, how do these aforementioned psychological vulnerabilities translate into the critical risk factors that facilitate deliberate firesetting and become the key clinical features observed in therapy? Within the M-TTAF, proximal factors and triggers represent important variables that interact with and reflect the psychological vulnerabilities of the individual. In brief, these variables relate to life events, contextual factors, internal affect or cognition, biological factors, and cultural factors that each individual experience throughout adulthood. Many of these factors could trigger or exacerbate existing psychological vulnerabilities. For example, experiencing a relationship breakdown (life event) is hypothesised to trigger or exacerbate self/emotional regulation issues and/or any pre-existing inappropriate fire-coping scripts. On the other hand, pre-existing psychological vulnerabilities in the form of poor coping (falling under the rubric of self/emotional regulation issues) may trigger the occurrence of stressful life events (e.g., financial issues, relationship breakdowns) that generate strong internal affect (e.g., hopelessness, frustration), creating a feedback loop that exacerbates pre-existing psychological vulnerabilities (i.e., poor coping and an inappropriate fire-coping script). Importantly, the interaction between psychological vulnerabilities and proximal factors and triggers is believed to be moderated by the two key factors of mental health and self-esteem. For example, poor mental health and self-esteem are hypothesised to exacerbate the development of negative effects resulting from proximal factors and triggers influencing psychological vulnerabilities. Once psychological vulnerabilities have been triggered or exacerbated, they become what are called "critical risk factors" that result in attempted or actual deliberate firesetting. Within the M-TTAF, it is possible for an individual to hold vulnerabilities to set fires (e.g., fire interest) and yet never set or attempt to set a deliberate fire. This is because their psychological vulnerability never reaches the critical threshold of being propelled into critical risk factors (i.e., the appropriate synergies between vulnerabilities, proximal factors, and moderators never occur). Within the M-TTAF, cognition and affect experienced at the time of and following the firesetting are conceptualised as being important factors for determining whether or not firesetting behaviour becomes reinforced and repetitive (see Jackson et al., 1987 or Fineman, 1980, 1995). However, the M-TTAF also recognises that individuals can desist from firesetting themselves either naturally (e.g., via identity change) or via rehabilitation (e.g., the Fire Intervention Programme for Prisoners, Gannon, 2012, 2017; the Firesetting Intervention Programme for Mentally Disordered Offenders, Gannon & Lockerbie, 2011, 2012, 2014, 2017).

Tier 2 of the M-TTAF (Table 3.1) specifies five example subtypes or "trajectories" of those who set fires according to the predicted clusters of critical risk factors within Tier 1 of the M-TTAF. The five key subtypes presented are antisocial, grievance, fire interest, emotionally expressive or need for recognition, and multi-faceted. The *antisocial* subtype describes individuals with the prominent critical risk factor of offence-supportive attitudes or values supporting general criminality. These individuals are also described as being likely to hold self-regulation problems in the form of poor impulse control and as being predominately male. Here, individuals may have an extensive criminal record that began at an early age and may also have attracted an adult diagnosis of antisocial personality disorder (American Psychiatric Association [APA], 2013). Thus, firesetting may have been used to achieve numerous antisocial goals (e.g., crime concealment, profit) and is hypothesised to be chosen as a criminal tool due to convenience. The grievance subtype refers to individuals with the prominent critical risk factor of self-regulation issues (i.e., relating to anger). Such individuals may also hold problems with their communication (i.e., low levels of assertiveness) and may set fires for revenge or retribution purposes. Here, fire may be the chosen tool of choice purely due to convenience or as a result of an inappropriate fire script relating to their personal experience with fire (i.e., of fire being dangerous and fear invoking; the *aggression-fire fusion script*). The *fire interest* subtype refers to individuals with the prominent risk factor of inappropriate fire interest or scripts. These individuals are also likely to hold some fire specific offence-supportive attitudes (e.g., that the fire is controllable), and fires are set for sensory excitement or as a result of stress. The *emotionally expressive or need for recognition* subtype refers to individuals whose most prominent critical risk factor lies in the area of communication problems. There are two relevant subtypes noted based upon the presence of a further critical risk factor in the area of self-regulation. The emotionally expressive subtype is *unable* to self-regulate and so may use fire in an attempt to self-harm, suicide, or elicit help from others. This trajectory is likely to be associated with females and is likely to be associated with borderline personality disorder (see Coid, 1993; Coid et al., 1999; Miller & Fritzon, 2007). The need for recognition subtype, on the other hand, is a *highly effective* self-regulator who misuses fire due to the need for social recognition and

Table 3.1 The Original and Updated M-TTAF Trajectories: Tier 2[a]

Trajectory	Prominent Risk Factor	Other Likely Risk Factors	Potential Clinical Features	Potential Motivators
Antisocial	Offence-supportive attitudes and values (supporting general criminality)	Self-regulation issues (e.g., poor emotional modulation) Inappropriate fire script (e.g., fire destroy evidence script)	Antisocial values and attitudes Implusivity Conduct disorder or antisocial personality disorder	Vandalism or boredom Crime concealment Profit Revenge or retribution
Grievance	Self-regulation issues	Communication Problems Inappropriate fire script (e.g., fire-aggression fusion script)	Low assertiveness Poor communication Fire-aggression fusion script Anger (rumination) Hostility	Revenge or retribution
Fire interest	Inappropriate fire interest Inappropriate fire script (e.g., fire destroys evidence script)	Offence-supportive attitudes (supporting firesetting)	Fire fascination or interest Impulsivity Attitudes supporting fire	Fire interest or thrill Stress or boredom
Emotionally expressive or need for recognition	Communication problems	Self-regulation issues[b] (e.g., poor emotional modulation) Inappropriate fire script (e.g., fire is a powerful messenger of distress)[b]	Poor Communication Impulsivity Depression Fire-coping fusion script Personality traits or disorder	Cry for help[b] Self-harm[b] Suicide[b] Need for Recognition
Multi-faceted	Offence-supportive attitudes or values (supporting general criminality and firesetting) Inappropriate fire interest Inappropriate fire script (e.g., fire-aggression fusion script)	Self-regulation issues Communication problems	Pervasive firesetting or general criminal behaviour Fire fascination or interest Antisocial values or attitudes Conduct disorder or antisocial personality disorder	Various

[a]Minor additions to Tier 2 are underlined.
[b]Emotionally expressive subtype only.

approval which is not communicated appropriately (i.e., the hero firesetter). It is hypothesised that this subtype may hold personality problems in the form of narcissism that drive and reinforce a need for social recognition. Finally, the *multi-faceted* subtype refers to individuals characterised by the two prominent critical risk factors of offence-supportive attitudes supporting criminal behaviour and inappropriate fire interest or scripts. These individuals may also hold critical risk factors in the areas of self-regulation and communication problems and are likely to hold antisocial personality disorder (APA, 2013). Such individuals are hypothesised to be largely male and to misuse fire pervasively in the service of any goal as a result of their antisocial attitudes and fire interest.

The M-TTAF was constructed using empirical research related to both males and females who have set fires. Since its development in 2012, it has received some empirical support for the Tier 2 trajectories from researchers independent from the model developers (i.e., empirical adequacy; see Campbell, 2016; Dalhuisen et al., 2017; Long et al., 2014; Nanayakkara et al., 2020a). The M-TTAF attempts to explain all of the possible motivators associated with firesetting and incorporates many complex mechanisms, theories, and assumptions. Consequently, the M-TTAF holds some weaknesses in the areas of *explanatory depth* and theoretical *coherence*. Nevertheless, it combines previously isolated theories and literatures with empirical research relating to firesetting (i.e., knitting together parts of the FAT, script theory, and DBT) illustrating theoretical *unification*. The M-TTAF appears to hold substantial *clinical fertility* due to the description of particular trajectories or subtypes of individuals who set fires (i.e., Tier 2) and the description of their key clinical features. In fact, the M-TTAF has been used to guide assessment and direct clinical resources in established treatment programmes for deliberate firesetting (e.g., ACART; Fritzon et al., 2013 and Firesetting Intervention Programme for Prisoners (FIPP); Gannon, 2012, 2017).

Refreshing the M-TTAF

Although the M-TTAF is only a decade old at the time of writing this book, research and clinical knowledge of firesetting have accumulated substantially over this period. In light of this, there are a small number of areas in the M-TTAF that we would like to update. We have also noted in many of our training courses on firesetting that practitioners ask us about how personality disorder fits within Tier 1, illustrating some issues with the M-TTAF's theoretical *depth* and *coherence*. Thus, in this part of the chapter, we attempt to refresh particular aspects of the theory in order to further improve the *empirical adequacy, depth, unification, coherence,* and *fertility* of the M-TTAF. We would like to emphasise that in no way are we attempting to amend the core elements or mechanisms of the model in any sense. We still recommend interested readers refer to the original M-TTAF article by Gannon and colleagues (2012) to learn in detail about this key theory. However, we also recommend that the current book chapter is consulted to gather the latest supplementary information.

Overall, there are two key elements of the M-TTAF (Tier 1) that we would like to update which relate to the concepts of (1) fire scripts and (2) personality disorder as well as three minor diagrammatical changes relating to the concepts of psychological vulnerabilities, critical risk factors, and reinforcement. On the basis of these changes, we then provide updates to Tier 2.

Fire Scripts

In our original documentation of fire scripts in the M-TTAF, we refer only to the concept of *inappropriate* fire scripts. As we have conducted trainings on this aspect, however, we have realised that it was neglectful not to mention the fact that all of us will hold a script of some sort or other regarding fire. By script, we are referring to learnt cognition regarding how fire is viewed and utilised. Many of us have learnt an *appropriate* fire script that views fire as "cosy" and appropriately stimulating in certain contexts (e.g., a log fire, candle, or bonfire night). Within this script, fire is deemed to be safe and pleasant as long as it is treated safely and respectfully.

When the learned script is an inappropriate one, however, it can lead to fire being misused extensively even when an individual is not necessarily interested in fire. As noted earlier, work has now been conducted to both describe and empirically examine fire-specific scripts in relation to firesetting since the advent of the original M-TTAF (see Butler, 2018; Butler & Gannon, 2015). This has highlighted two particular scripts not mentioned in the original M-TTAF: *fire is a powerful messenger of distress*, and *fire is the best way to destroy evidence*. For clarity purposes, we would like to add these two scripts into the M-TTAF so as to extend the repertoire of scripts from the existing two (i.e., *fire-coping, fire-aggression fusion*) to four scripts. The additional two scripts are important since they are able to explain how firesetting might come to be used as a preferred tool to elicit attention (i.e., the *fire as a powerful messenger of distress* script) or cover up another crime (i.e., *the fire is the best way to destroy evidence* script) *in the absence* of fire interest. The former script refers to fire having been learnt to be a powerful messenger of *distress* (e.g., to elicit attention or cry for help). Presumably, this script may be learnt via social learning, which suggests that early experiences with fire have a direct impact on fire script formation. This script differs from the fire-coping script since it refers uniquely to fire being used to communicate distress rather than a general coping mechanism to be used across various situations. The script regarding the destruction of evidence refers to an inappropriate script regarding the use of fire that has evolved through criminal behaviour engagement (either as a child or an adult). Here, fire has come to be a preferred method of destroying evidence via criminal experience and knowledge around the destructive nature of fire. This script is an important one that appears to solve the clinical puzzle regarding why some antisocial individuals appear to misuse fire repeatedly in the context of holding no discernible interest in fire. In the original M-TTAF, we presented fire misuse by antisocial individuals as being dependent upon fire being convenient. And for some individuals, this may be the case. However, the *fire is the best way to destroy evidence* script explains *preferential* misuse of fire by these individuals.

Through incorporating the latest single-factor theory and research on inappropriate fire scripts into the M-TTAF, we believe that we have strengthened the key areas of *empirical adequacy, depth, unification, coherence,* and ultimately *clinical fertility*. Knowing that the M-TTAF incorporates the latest findings and theory in relation to fire scripts ensures that there is a clearer account of why particular individuals misuse fire which is of clear value for more accurate assessment and targeted intervention attempts.

Personality Disorders

In the original M-TTAF, personality disorders are referred to only in Tier 2. This has led to some professionals questioning where in Tier 1 such personality disorders would be located.

In other words, the M-TTAF appeared to have problems in the areas of theoretical *depth* and *coherence*. Personality disorders can be defined as pervasive and developmental conditions that impact an individual's cognition, affect, and functioning/ behaviour such that they differ markedly from others within their culture (see DSM-5; APA, 2013). Within *Diagnostic and Statistical Manual of Mental Disorders*, fifth edition (DSM-5), personality disorders are grouped according to three clusters (see APA, 2013; Mayo Clinic, 2016). *Cluster A* personality disorders refer to paranoid personality, schizoid, and schizotypal personality disorders. These personality disorders are generally characterised by odd and unusual thoughts about others as well as eccentric thoughts and behaviours. *Cluster B* personality disorders refer to antisocial, borderline, histrionic, and narcissistic personality disorders. These personality disorders tend to be characterised by impulsive and unstable functioning or behaviour as well as striking and highly changeable affect. *Cluster C* personality disorders refer to avoidant, dependent, and obsessive-compulsive personality disorders. Here, the thoughts and functioning of the individual are generally characterised by anxiety and fear.

Personality disorders are generally believed to develop as a result of an—as yet—unknown combination of childhood adversity factors and genetic influences (Karterud & Kongerslev, 2019; Reichborn-Kjennerud et al., 2015; Ruocco & Carcone, 2016; Skoglund et al., 2019), and such disorders are commonly linked to firesetting (Ducat et al., 2013a; Gannon & Pina, 2010; Nanayakkara et al., 2020a; Ó Ciardha et al., 2015a). In the area of firesetting, Cluster B traits and disorders appear to have garnered significant support (Ducat et al., 2013a; Ó Ciardha et al., 2015a), particularly in females who have set fires (Nanayakkara et al., 2020a). Within the revised M-TTAF, personality disorders and traits are hypothesised to develop within the developmental context as a result of genetic inheritance, neurobiology, and environmental factors relating to the caregiver environment and learning experiences (Porter et al., 2020; Ruocco & Carcone, 2016; Skoglund et al., 2019). For example, in the case of borderline personality disorder, an individual who holds a greater genetic risk of developing this disorder (i.e., heritability; see Chanen & McCutcheon, 2013), whose early environment is characterised by chronic stress and abusive experiences, is likely to experience changes to their brain functioning during a period of increased brain development sensitivity. These neurological changes are hypothesised to result in the symptoms of borderline personality disorder (e.g., unstable affect, impulsivity, intense, pervasive self-harm attempts and suicidal behaviour, unstable interpersonal relationships) that are likely to emerge as vulnerabilities in the areas of self/emotional regulation issues and communication problems.

Through providing readers with further information regarding how the M-TTAF can account for the development of personality disorder within its framework, we hope that we have strengthened the key areas of *empirical depth, coherence*, and *clinical fertility*. Knowing how personality disorder fits within the structure of the M-TTAF ensures that clinicians hold a clearer and more coherent account of how personality disorder becomes a key psychological vulnerability that can play a role in firesetting.

Minor Diagrammatical Changes to Tier 1

An updated version of Tier 1 of the M-TTAF may be found in Figure 3.3. Compared with the original M-TTAF, three key areas of amendment are highlighted via underlined text or

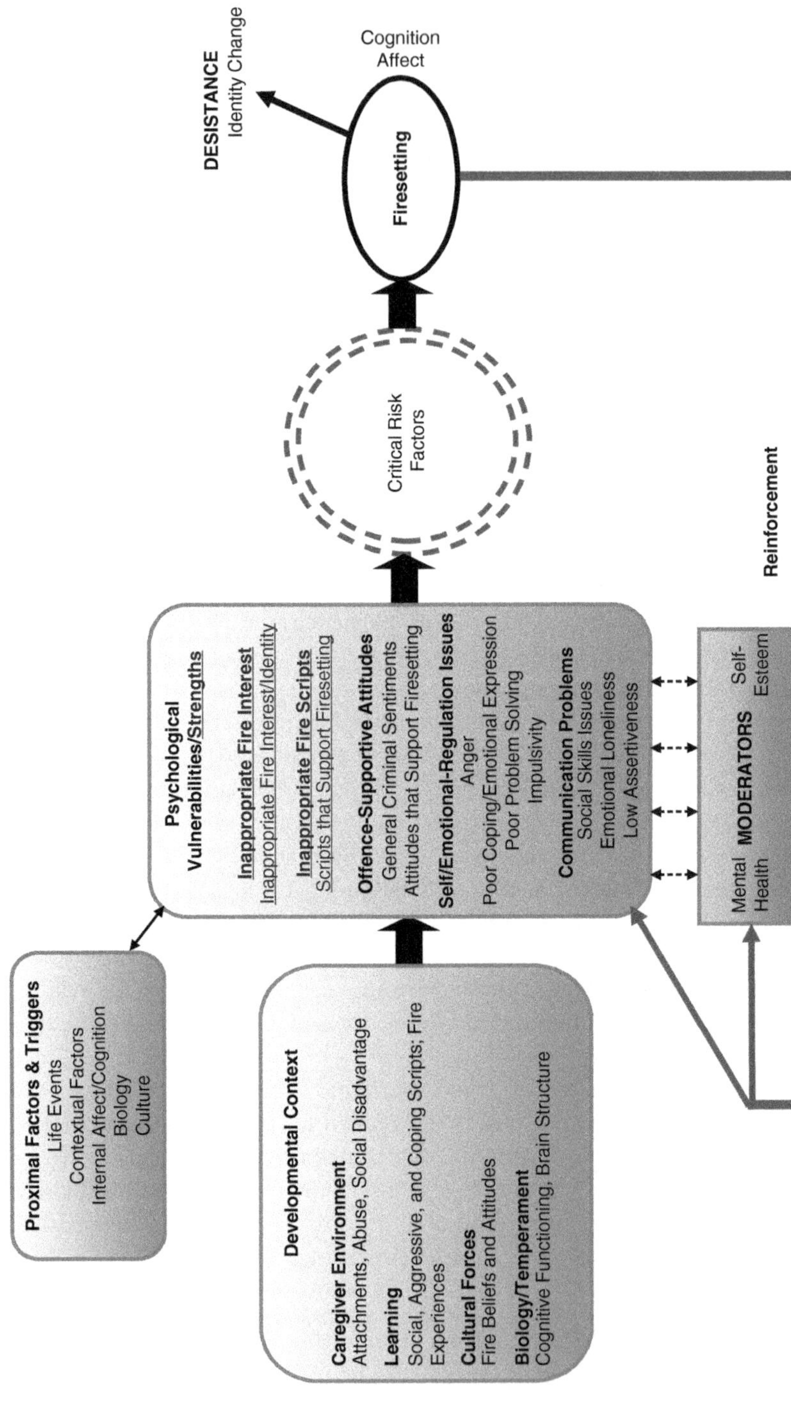

Figure 3.3 The updated M-TTAF: Tier 1 (adapted from Gannon et al., 2012).

broken lines. First, in the area of psychological vulnerabilities, we have amended the title of this section to read "Psychological Vulnerabilities and Strengths." We believe that this descriptor better describes the *combination* of psychological factors that each person will possess at this stage. Most certainly, for example, individuals will hold a suite of both psychological vulnerabilities and strengths. Highlighting the aspect of strengths is useful since it enables clinicians to search for these and view them as potential factors of risk (e.g., highly regulated planning) or protection (e.g., good communication skills) according to each individual's unique formulation. Within the suite of factors presented in the psychological vulnerabilities and strengths box, we have also separated out the concept of inappropriate fire scripts from inappropriate fire interest. At this time, we think it is appropriate to present inappropriate fire scripts separately given the theory and research that has now developed to support this concept. In the previous M-TTAF, presenting scripts in combination with fire interest may have been confusing and given readers the impression that fire interest always co-occurred with inappropriate fire scripts.

The second area of amendment relates to the diagrammatical depiction of critical risk factors in the model. Here, we have updated this element—now depicted by a cycle—to make it visually clearer that a particular combination of psychological vulnerabilities and strengths reach the critical threshold of being propelled into critical risk factors prior to a firesetting offence occurring.

Finally, the third area of amendment relates to the depiction of firesetting reinforcement. In the M-TTAF, cognition and affect experienced at the time of and following the firesetting are conceptualised as being important factors for determining whether or not firesetting behaviour becomes reinforced and repetitive (see Jackson et al., 1987 or Fineman, 1980, 1995). Here, reinforcement principles are hypothesised to explain repetitive firesetting. For example, an individual who experiences significant pride and positive affect from misusing fire is likely to repeat firesetting in pursuit of these positive cognitions and affect. However, similar to Jackson et al.'s (1987) FAT principles, negative consequences of fire such as social rejection and punishment are hypothesised to further exacerbate pre-existing psychological vulnerabilities or strengths that led to the firesetting behaviour in the first place. In other words, the individual's propensity to set fires becomes strengthened. In the original M-TTAF (see Figure 3.2), the reinforcement arrow erroneously points towards moderators, which is misleading for readers and may give the impression that there is something about these moderators, in particular, that is being reinforced. While such moderators can become reinforced, so, too, can the psychological strengths and vulnerabilities.

In making each of these diagrammatical amendments, we have sought to provide a clearer and more coherent diagrammatical account of the variables and mechanisms associated with firesetting behaviour (i.e., increased theoretical coherence).

Changes to Tier 2

In light of the amendments made to Tier 1 of the M-TTAF, we have made some amendments to Tier 2. This relates to the antisocial trajectory, which in the original M-TTAF is presented without any mention of scripts. While we believe it is possible for antisocial trajectory individuals to set fires simply because fire is conveniently to hand, based on Butler and Gannon's (2015) work and our clinical work with individuals who have set fires, we now hypothesise that scripts are likely to be evident for this subtype. In particular, for example, we would expect the *fire is a best way to destroy evidence script* to be evident for individuals who set fires to conceal crimes, and the *fire-aggression fusion script* to be evident for individuals who set fires out of revenge or retribution. Furthermore, within the emotionally expressive trajectory, we would also expect such individuals to hold the critical risk factor of *fire is a powerful messenger of distress* in addition to or in place of the *fire-coping script*. Based on Butler and Gannon's (2015) work, we have also provided examples of the scripts likely to be held by the subtypes already noted in Tier 2. These minor additions to Tier 2 have been added in underlined text to Figure 3.1.

Unidentified Trajectories

There have been occasions, during our training and individual clinical practice, when we have come across individuals who have set fires who do not easily fit into the trajectories offered into Tier 2. We view this situation as inevitable since the key trajectories are intended simply to be "guides" for consulting clinicians, and firesetting is a complex behaviour that will not always fit neatly into preassigned categories. For example, we have found in our own practice that firesetting that appears to have occurred as a result of intense peer pressure does not always fit satisfactorily into the pre-defined Tier 2 trajectories. When this occurs, it is critical that consulting clinicians do not try to force fit individuals into the Tier 2 trajectories. Instead, what is required is expert formulation using Tier 1 of the M-TTAF as a guide whilst weaving in the individual aspects of the case.

Conclusions, Ways of Working, and Future Directions

Encouraging progress has been made over the past decade or so in terms of our theoretical understanding of firesetting. First, typological explanations of firesetting have moved beyond simplistic and subjective classifications to more objective and sophisticated methods (e.g., crime scene profiling, Canter & Fritzon, 1998; Kocsis & Cooksey, 2002; cluster analysis techniques, Nanayakkara et al., 2020a, 2020b). Second, the development of the M-TTAF has knitted together the strengths of previously popular theories of firesetting (i.e., Jackson et al.'s [1987] FAT and Fineman's [1995] DBT) into one overarching multifactor theory of firesetting that is able to account for firesetting that occurs in the absence of fire interest, firesetting in the context of poor mental health (including personality disorder), and both male- and female-perpetrated firesetting. Related to this, we have seen the development of a significant single-factor theory of firesetting (i.e., inappropriate firesetting scripts) that is able to explain why someone would repeatedly set fires in the absence of fire interest (see Butler, 2018; Butler & Gannon, 2015). Finally, researchers have developed micro-process theories to explain how the offence process is likely to unfold for individuals who set fires (see Barnoux et al., 2015; Tyler et al., 2014).

Thus, professionals working in this area now hold the theoretical resources necessary to engage in theoretically informed assessment and treatment practices. For example, practitioners tasked with assessing adults who have set fires can use the updated M-TTAF to structure their assessments and lines of enquiry to make them as comprehensive as possible. Individuals tasked with treating individuals who have set fires can also use this theory alongside the information on inappropriate fire scripts to ensure that appropriate individuals receive firesetting treatment (e.g., antisocial trajectory individuals who hold inappropriate fire scripts) and steer their intervention towards targeted and effective ways of reducing firesetting (i.e., targeting the scripts that are leading to repeated fire use; see Gannon, 2012, 2017). Importantly, the micro-process theories developed (Barnoux et al., 2015; Tyler et al., 2014) emphasise the importance of examining childhood experiences with fire during assessment and treatment processes so as to understand how these experiences have fed into decisions to misuse fire later in adulthood.

Despite these developments, there is still theoretical work to be conducted in the area of firesetting. The M-TTAF and its amendments require further concerted external evaluations. Furthermore, it is critical to continue research activity into promising single factors that may feed into more comprehensive theories such as the M-TTAF. For example, further work is needed to examine how fire interest and scripts are developed and how these factors interrelate to other key variables implicated in firesetting. Further work is also needed in the area of offence-supportive attitudes to aid our understanding of which attitudes are likely to be important in firesetting.

There is no doubt that practitioners working in this area need to ensure that they are familiar with the latest available theory of firesetting as it continues to unfold. Contemporary theoretical developments indicate that firesetting is a complex criminal behaviour that requires expert and individualised formulation of a number of key variables. In the following chapter, we examine how the latest theoretical developments in firesetting can be used to aid best practice risk assessments for this client group.

4

Conducting Best Practice Risk Assessments in Deliberate Firesetting

Articulating the parameters in which a person is most likely to reoffend is one of the crucial functions of forensic clinical practice (Sturmey & McMurran, 2011). Typically, the primary aims of risk assessment are to answer two key questions: (1) under what circumstances did the offence occur? and (2) is the person likely to reoffend without any intervention? As will be discussed in this chapter, risk assessment protocols have also evolved to answer a third fundamental question: (3) what are the practical steps for managing risk of reoffending? Risk assessments enable the criminal justice system to effectively prioritise financial and human resources. They aid decision-making regarding length of custody and/or community supervision as well as placement on rehabilitation programmes and interventions (Bonta & Wormith, 2013).

Deliberate firesetting is commonly associated with preconceptions of high levels of recidivism. For example, people who set fires are a difficult group to resettle back into the community relative to individuals who have committed other types of offences (Allender et al., 2005). This is because a history of deliberate firesetting or arson is typically an exclusion criterion across the housing sector (e.g., Ellison et al., 2013). Residential managers are reluctant to approve accommodation applications due to perceived risk of further firesetting and damage or destruction of their property. An evidence-based risk assessment represents one way of attempting to re-assure these residential managers and allied professionals that risk of future firesetting has been adequately assessed so that any possible risk of firesetting is recognised early and managed appropriately.

This chapter first provides an overview of the literature on baseline firesetting recidivism rates. In other words, how likely is it that someone with a pre-existing firesetting offence will reoffend using fire again? The latest research examining static and dynamic risk factors associated with repeat firesetting is then discussed to provide insight into the possible predictors of firesetting recidivism. Following this, the small array of published and unpublished risk assessments available for use with individuals who have set fires are presented, concluding with a guide to conducting a firesetting risk assessment using the Multi-Trajectory Theory of Adult Firesetting (M-TTAF; Gannon et al., 2012; see Chapter 3).

Adult Deliberate Firesetting: Theory, Assessment, and Treatment, First Edition. Theresa A. Gannon, Nichola Tyler, Caoilte Ó Ciardha and Emma Alleyne.
© 2022 John Wiley & Sons Ltd. Published 2022 by John Wiley & Sons Ltd.

Prevalence of Firesetting Recidivism

Despite the apparent perception that firesetting recidivism is high, the prevalence rates tell a somewhat different story. The research on firesetting recidivism varies depending on: (1) the definition of recidivism used (e.g., prosecuted versus non-prosecuted incidents), (2) the type of data (self-report versus official records), (3) the samples examined (psychiatric versus prison samples), and (4) the study designs (e.g., retrospective versus prospective). For example, Rice and Harris (1996) conducted a prospective study (a rare occurrence in the firesetting literature) in which they identified 243 men in a maximum security psychiatric institution who had engaged in firesetting. During the follow-up period of approximately 7.8 years, 208 men had an opportunity to reoffend, of whom 16% set a subsequent fire. Firesetting recidivism, in this study, was defined as any charge (arson or otherwise) when firesetting had been documented as part of the offence.

More recently, there have been retrospective studies that define firesetting recidivism as having been formally charged for a subsequent arson offence (Ducat et al., 2015; Edwards & Grace, 2013). These studies capture people who recidivate regardless of the forensic setting (i.e., prison, psychiatric, community settings), but the results are limited to the specific charge of arson. As a result, reported recidivism rates are much lower (i.e., 6.2% after 10 year follow-up [Edwards & Grace, 2013]; 5.3% after 6.9 year follow-up [Ducat et al., 2015]).

What is important to also note is that people who set fires are not necessarily specialists in their reoffending. It is more likely that they commit other types of offending behaviour (Soothill et al., 2004). As mentioned previously, Rice and Harris (1996) found that 16% of their participants committed subsequent fires on follow-up, but nearly a third (31%) committed a subsequent violent offence, and more than half (57%) committed a subsequent nonviolent offence. These findings have been echoed in more recent studies (see Ducat et al., 2015).

Clinicians need a clear base rate of reoffending (firesetting and other offending alike) to inform their decision-making regarding the content and intensity of a risk management plan. To date, the most rigorous examination of firesetting recidivism has been a meta-analysis by Sambrooks et al. (2021). In their study, they were able to analyse data across 25 samples ($N = 12{,}294$). They scrutinised the data by accounting for definitional disparities, type and source of data, and study designs and only included studies that had an identifiable sample of individuals who had not been treated specifically for their firesetting behaviour. The base rate of firesetting reoffending defined as an officially recorded criminal arson was found to be 8%–10%. When analysing data that used a broader definition of firesetting, however, the firesetting reoffending rate was 17%–20%. More important, people with a history of setting fires were five times more likely to set subsequent fires relative to individuals with no firesetting history. In addition to firesetting reoffending, Sambrooks et al. (2021) found that up to two thirds (57%–66%) of people with a history of setting fires subsequently offended in other ways.

These base rates highlight two key messages. First, it is fundamental for clinicians to account for definitional and source discrepancies when conducting and writing up risk assessments. Second, base rates for firesetting and general offending behaviour suggest that a history of firesetting warrants the attention of clinicians when conducting risk assessments and developing risk management plans.

Risk and Protective Factors: The Basis for Assessment

To assess the likelihood an individual will re-offend, we must have a clear understanding of the key factors that increase and mitigate this risk. Bonta and Andrews (2017), as major proponents of rehabilitation theory, conceptualised the process of rehabilitation to consist of three core principles: (1) *risk*—the criminal justice response should match individual levels of risk to reoffend; (2) *need*—the response, in the form of treatment, should target the criminogenic needs identified in assessment; and (3) *responsivity*—the treatment programme or rehabilitation intervention should be tailored to individual attributes, abilities, and motivations to maximise effectiveness (i.e., the risk-need-responsivity [RNR] model). To predict "risk" of reoffending (first principle), Bonta and Andrews (2017) advocated for developing an evidence base of the static and dynamic risk factors that best predict the problem behaviour. *Static risk factors* are typically historical events that shape a person's character and disposition (Douglas & Skeem, 2005; Eisenberg et al., 2019). For example, past behaviour is a good predictor of future behaviour. If someone has previously offended, the likelihood they will reoffend is higher than someone who has never offended. Such factors tell us a lot about what a person experienced, and as a result, what they might be predisposed to do; however, the factors themselves are not changeable.

Criminogenic needs (also known as dynamic risk factors) can be defined as modifiable features of an individual and/or their environment that are associated with their reoffending (Heffernan & Ward, 2017). It is vital to highlight the changeable nature of these features because in addition to predicting risk, criminogenic needs are fundamental to the process of attenuating risk. That is, the key aim of any form of treatment is to influence features of a person (or their circumstances) that result in an outcome of behaviour change and ultimately reduce risk of reoffending (Kroner & Yessine, 2013). Further, it is important to understand the extent to which influencing change will require higher versus lower intensity interventions. For example, a person's personality (an enduring characteristic) is typically a stable feature that is resistant yet not impossible to change. If a personality characteristic is identified as a contributing factor to offending behaviour, then it is likely a more intensive form of treatment would be required to effect lasting change. Alternatively, some dynamic risk factors can be characterised as acute and rapidly changing (e.g., substance abuse). Such factors need attention but perhaps not as intensive and long term to achieve the desired treatment shifts. Ultimately, these factors (whether stable or acute; Hanson & Harris, 2001) are ideal targets for treatment given their malleability.

Bonta and Andrews (2017) posited that the following "central eight" risk or needs factors (second principle) are likely predictors of criminal behaviour (note all but one are dynamic risk factors): (1) history of antisocial behaviour (static), (2) antisocial attitudes, (3) antisocial peers, (4) antisocial personality, (5) family or marital factors, (6) lack of achievement in education or employment, (7) lack of prosocial leisure activities, and (8) substance abuse. When assessing risk of future offending, these types of factors warrant specific attention.

Finally, *protective factors* have been more recently highlighted as key to risk assessment. Their inclusion form part of a movement from a deficits-based approach to a strengths-based approach to rehabilitation. Protective factors can act as buffers from unavoidable risk factors and as a result have a risk-reducing effect on offending (de Vogel et al., 2009). They also have a dual function of increasing the predictive accuracy of risk assessments while contributing to a more well rounded clinical case formulation (Serin et al., 2016). The inclusion of protective factors in developing risk management plans also enhances clients' responsivity (Bonta & Andrews' [2017] third principle) because clients are more likely to be motivated to engage in work that is framed towards positive life outcomes (de Vries Robbé & Willis, 2017). Ultimately, the aim of risk assessment is to present a complete picture that includes both risk and protective factors, consisting of historical or contextual structure as well as current or changeable features to aid forensic clinical decision-making.

Risk and Protective Factors for Repeat Firesetting

To develop guidance on conducting a firesetting risk assessment, there must first be a review of the research on firesetting recidivism and risk factors. Recidivism research, to date, has provided evidence for static and historical factors, whereby socio-demographic characteristics associated with repeat firesetting include being male (Ducat et al., 2015), single (Dickens et al., 2009; Rice & Harris, 1996), unemployed (Dickens et al., 2009), younger at the time of their first ever firesetting offence (Dickens et al., 2009; Ducat et al., 2015), and younger at the time of their first ever offence of any kind (Ducat et al., 2015; Field, 2016). Individuals who engage in repeat firesetting, compared with one-time firesetting, are characterised by adverse childhood experiences such as chaotic or disruptive family environments (Dickens et al., 2009; Doley, 2009; Rice & Harris, 1991), poor school attainment (Dickens et al., 2009; Doley, 2009; Rice & Harris, 1991), and externalising behavioural issues (Field, 2016). Their offending history is typically quite extensive (Barnett & Spitzer, 1994; Doley, 2009; Ducat et al., 2015) and varied, involving offences such as firesetting (Ducat et al., 2015; Edwards & Grace, 2013; Koson & Dvoskin, 1982; Rice & Harris, 1996; Sapsford et al., 1978) and property offences (Doley, 2009; Edwards & Grace, 2013; Field, 2016). However, it appears that a history of violent offending is not associated with subsequent firesetting (Rice & Harris, 1996).

Further static factors include the unique features of the *modus operandi* identified within the case files for those who perpetrate multiple fires. The fires are typically ignited during the weekend (Rice & Harris, 1996), within the vicinity of the perpetrator's own home, and usually the target is a building rather than other types of objects (Repo et al., 1997). Crucially, firesetting recidivism has not been associated with setting fires characterised as *dangerous* (i.e., increased probability of harm to others; Dickens et al., 2009). Essentially, the evidence suggests that the severity of a firesetting incident is not indicative of future firesetting behaviour and would not have predictive value in a risk assessment. However, it is important to note that people who set multiple fires are less likely to make attempts to extinguish the fire than people who have only set one fire (Wyatt et al., 2019). Finally, firesetting recidivism is associated with acting alone (Field, 2016; Rice & Harris, 1996) rather than in the company of others.

Firesetting recidivism has also been associated with greater levels of past engagement with mental health services. In reviewing clinical histories, people who engage in repeat firesetting appear more likely to have had contact with psychiatric services during childhood and adolescence (Ducat et al., 2015; Field, 2016) and have a diagnostic history consisting of personality disorder (Dickens et al., 2009; Repo et al., 1997; Rice & Harris, 1996; Wyatt et al., 2019), psychotic disorder (Ducat et al., 2015; Lindberg et al., 2005), and/ or substance misuse (Ducat et al., 2015; Koson & Dvoskin, 1982; Lindberg et al., 2005; Repo et al., 1997). However, whether or not these diagnoses were implicated in the firesetting incidents remains unclear. It is also important to note that repeat firesetting has not been associated with clinical diagnoses of depression and anxiety (Ducat et al., 2015).

The literature on dynamic risk factors and their link to firesetting recidivism is not as extensive as what has been discussed for static factors. There is some evidence of a link between the presence of an inappropriate interest or fascination in fire and repeat fireset-ting (Dickens et al., 2009; Rice & Harris, 1996). An inappropriate interest in fire may mani-fest itself via extensive observation of fire, an attraction to or curiosity for fire paraphernalia, and/or the peripheral experience of the firesetting context (e.g., observing others' reac-tions). Fire interest has also been found to develop from early childhood (Del Bove & Mackay, 2011; Dickens et al., 2009; Rice & Harris, 1996; Soothill & Pope, 1973). Additional psychological factors implicated in repeat firesetting include aggression-related attitudes (Rice & Harris, 1996), impulsivity (Wyatt et al., 2019), and relational issues characterised by poor interpersonal skills (Field, 2016).

Although the research on dynamic risk factors is sparce, there are cross-sectional, com-parative studies that have highlighted factors that distinguish people who set fires from others in similar circumstances (e.g., serving prison sentences for other types of offending) but with no firesetting history. These studies offer likely targets for treatment (i.e., crimino-genic needs) that would otherwise be neglected in generic intervention programmes. For example, the relational issues already identified could be explained by deficits in commu-nication skills and assertiveness (Jackson et al., 1987; Noblett & Nelson, 2001; Rice & Harris, 2008) in addition to high impulsivity (Räsänen et al., 1996), as seen in the wider firesetting literature. Further criminogenic needs include problems with emotion regula-tion (Gannon et al., 2013; Rix, 1994), maladaptive coping (Dickens et al., 2012), fire safety awareness (Gannon et al., 2013), and fire-related scripts (i.e., *fire is a powerful messenger*, Butler & Gannon, 2021). The roles these factors play in recurrent firesetting are not fully substantiated; however, their relationships with firesetting behaviour offer insight into why a person uses fire in their offending and how engrained these attitudes and beliefs are. Further, their ability to distinguish people who set fires from those who offend in other ways suggests that targeting them in treatment could lead to effective behaviour change. For example, a person who holds an inappropriate fire script should be concerning to the clinician conducting a risk assessment because extant literature has evidenced the link between deep-rooted offence-supportive cognition and (re)offending (e.g., sexual offend-ing; Hanson & Morton-Bougon, 2005).

Very little research has focused on protective factors in relation to firesetting. There are, however, inferences that can be made from the findings of existing studies. For example, it appears that individuals who set fires are not likely to have a learning disability (Sambrooks et al., 2021). This suggests that cognitive ability could be used as a platform for pursuing educational and/or employment opportunities. Similarly, Gannon et al. (2012) theorised that high self-esteem could act as a buffer from the effects of triggers interacting with an individual's psychological vulnerabilities. Further protective factors can come to fruition as a result of treatment engagement, as theorised in the M-TTAF.

However, it is important to note that this is an area that requires robust empirical research to form the evidence base for clinical formulations. As it stands, there is very little evidence to draw from.

Risk Assessment Protocols

There has been an evolution of the process and format of risk assessment protocols and tools. The *first generation* of risk assessment relied solely on the professional judgement of the clinician conducting the assessment (Bonta & Andrews, 2017). However, decision-making was not based on the latest developments in research, so this approach fell out of favour. The desire for an evidence-based approach to risk assessment birthed *second-generation* risk assessment tools that utilised actuarial algorithms. In short, actuarial tools assign quantitative scores to risk factors that have been shown to increase risk of reoffending (Kim et al., 2008). Actuarial tools have demonstrated superior ability in the prediction of reoffending when compared with professional judgement (i.e., *first generation*; Andrews et al., 2006; Harris et al., 1993). However, these tools are typically reliant on historical, static risk factors (e.g., history of offending) and do not account for positive change (i.e., crime desistance). As a result, a person's "score," based on historical factors, will either stay the same or go up (if new factors are scored) but will never decrease because past experiences can not be revised nor excluded.

The shortcomings of actuarial methods led to the emergence of *third-generation* tools based on structured professional judgement (SPJ). Essentially, it became evident that for a risk assessment to be most informative, it needed to account for dynamic risk factors, in addition to the predictive value of static risk factors (Salo et al., 2019). As such, the dynamic and changeable nature of factors can be contextualised to inform risk management plans. Sensitivity to change is both paramount to predicting risk of reoffending (Raynor, 2007) and identifying treatment targets for intervention (Bonta & Andrews, 2017), which reaps greater reductions in reoffending when incorporated in intervention planning.

Firesetting Risk Assessment Tools

The likelihood for someone who has set a fire to reoffend in any way appears to be high given the existing base rates discussed previously. To date, a small number of published and unpublished tools have been designed to assess the likelihood of reoffending amongst individuals with a history of firesetting. These tools span second- and third-generation risk assessment types.

Predicting firesetting risk using static factors. In New Zealand, Edwards and Grace (2013) conducted a retrospective, 10-year follow-up study with a national sample of 1,250 individuals convicted of arson. The aim of their study was to produce an actuarial model of arson, violent, and nonviolent recidivism using accessible data on static variables. During the follow-up period, they found that 6.2% ($n = 77$) of their sample was convicted of a subsequent arson offence. This is in stark contrast to subsequent violent (48.5%; $n = 606$) and nonviolent (79.3%; $n = 991$) offending. Edwards and Grace (2013) were able to estimate predictive models for recidivism using forward stepwise Cox regressions and assessed their predictive validity in terms of the area under the receiver operating characteristic (ROC) curve (area under the curve [AUC]; Hosmer et al., 2013). They used data on socio-demographic characteristics, offence history (e.g., number of prior offences by offence type), and the details of the reference arson offence. Further, Edwards and Grace (2013) randomly divided their sample into two sub-samples: the developmental group (data analyses used to estimate the predictive model) and the validation group (data used to cross-validate the model).

The actuarial model for arson recidivism consisted of three significant predictors: (1) young age (i.e., younger than 18 years) at first arson (odds ratio [OR] = 2.51), (2) reference arson consisted of multiple fires (OR = 3.27), and (3) higher number of prior vandalism offences (OR = 1.41). When computing the area under the ROC curves (AUC), the value of the developmental group was 0.70, demonstrating acceptable discrimination (Hosmer et al., 2013) between those who did and did not commit a subsequent arson offence. The AUC value for the validation group was 0.68, indicating relatively stable predictive validity.

The findings from Edwards and Grace's (2013) study highlighted the importance of key static variables in assessing the likelihood of future firesetting. In particular, age of onset, prolific firesetting behaviour, and nonviolent offending history resulted in significant increases in the odds of repeat firesetting (but see Edwards, (2020) for a validation study that did not provide full support for Edwards and Grace's original actuarial model). The variable showing the most impact was prolific firesetting behaviour at time of index where individuals were 3.27 times more likely to set a subsequent fire. As discussed previously, these factors can inform initial decision-making regarding placement (e.g., community versus custody) and programming (e.g., need for intervention); however, an individual's risk level would remain unchanged without consideration of complementary dynamic risk factors that can shift with treatment.

Predicting firesetting risk using dynamic factors. To date, there has been a preference for third-generation risk assessment tools due to the dual function of case formulation (i.e., explaining how the various risk factors interact to produce firesetting behaviour) and risk management planning (Sturmey & McMurran, 2011). The Historical, Clinical, and Risk Management (HCR)-20 Version 3 (Douglas et al., 2013), based on SPJ principles, is the "gold standard" for violence risk assessment. This protocol guides an evidence-based evaluation of risk and treatment needs and has been well validated with prison and psychiatric samples (Strub et al., 2014). Given the paucity of fire-specific tools, the HCR-20 has been adopted by some clinicians to guide firesetting risk assessment. It is important to note, however, that the HCR-20 was designed to assess violence risk and was developed from extensive research on the factors associated with violent behaviour. Therefore, its remit for assessing risk of reoffending is limited to behaviours that involve actual and/or threatened violence. As such, past firesetting behaviour can be recorded within the HCR-20 framework as either historical violent offending (if the firesetting was underpinned by violent intentions) or historical antisocial behaviour. Either way, the utility of this information is to aid decision-making regarding future violent reoffending. The validity of using the HCR-20 to assess firesetting reoffending has neither been evaluated nor evidenced. Thus, it is only in the context of violence that the HCR-20 could be a valid assessment of firesetting. However, as previously mentioned, not all firesetting is motivated by violent intentions (e.g., financial gain, boredom, crime concealment; Gannon & Pina, 2010). Also, the

HCR-20 does not explicitly capture factors specific to firesetting such as firesetting history and offence characteristics, fire interest, and associated affective or cognitive factors (Gannon & Pina, 2010).

To address some of this gap, Long et al. (2013) developed the St. Andrew's Fire and Arson Risk Instrument (SAFARI). In line with SPJ principles (Hart et al., 2011), the SAFARI uses the Functional Analysis Framework (Jackson, 1994; Jackson et al., 1987; see Chapter 3 for further detail) to guide the type of information needed to produce an evidence-based clinical formulation. The protocol for conducting the firesetting risk assessment involves adapting the HCR-20 framework to capture supplementary data on (1) the types of scenarios when firesetting is likely to occur; (2) the cognitive, affective, and behavioural antecedents to the firesetting; and (3) the internal and/or external consequences of firesetting that reinforce use of fire (Long et al., 2013). In essence, the SAFARI augments the HCR-20 by guiding the data gathering phase to include fire-related information in addition to the violence risk information the HCR-20 was designed to capture. It benefits from knitting together a well-established violence risk literature and protocol, with a firesetting theoretical framework. Therefore, in instances when fire is used in the context of violence, the SAFARI improves upon the HCR-20 and may be a valid approach. However, this leaves clinicians with first having to identify the motivations of the firesetting prior to deciding which risk assessment tool to use.

An alternative to the SAFARI is Logan et al.'s (2010) *Fire-setting Risk Assessment and Management Worksheet*, which guides the clinician through a similar process as the HCR-20 (e.g., assessing presence and relevance of factors); however, there are key differences in the structure and nature of the factors. First, the collection of factors are not arranged into historical, clinical, and risk categories. Instead, Logan and colleagues (2010) drew on Weerasekera's (1996) 5Ps Model of clinical formulation (i.e., problem, predisposing, precipitating, perpetuating, and protective factors). The worksheet lists 16 predisposing (historical) factors and seven precipitating factors or triggers for clinicians to rate presence and relevance. Clinicians are guided towards identifying the key factors implicated in the firesetting behaviour as well as additional perpetuating and protective factors to produce the clinical risk formulation. These factors are then further conceptualised into risk scenarios to inform treatment planning.

Second, where the HCR-20 assesses violence histories and violence-related attitudes and beliefs, the firesetting worksheet assesses firesetting history and broadly defined antisocial attitudes and beliefs. This allows clinicians the flexibility to capture violent and non-violent firesetting. However, the factors included in the worksheet are not always derived from theory or research. For example, the worksheet asks clinicians to rate the presence and relevance of *sexual dysfunction*. To date, there has yet to be an empirical link to substantiate the inclusion of this factor (Ó Ciardha, 2015). Alternatively, there has been some research (described earlier in this chapter) to support the assessment of fire interest and fascination, yet these important factors are not included in the worksheet.

Both the SAFARI and the Fire-setting Risk Assessment and Management Worksheet benefit from adopting a familiar methodology (e.g., HCR-20) that can be seamlessly incorporated into clinical practice. However, in both cases, a note of caution is required for two reasons. First, there have been significant advancements in our understanding of firesetting cognition not currently accounted for in either tool. For example, the SAFARI is based on the functional analysis framework, which does not account for fire-related scripts.

Equally, the Fire-setting Worksheet has not been updated with these latest developments. Second, these tools have not yet been evaluated on their effectiveness in predicting and formulating a plan to attenuate risk.

One of the best known risk assessment tools in the literature is the Northgate Firesetter Risk Assessment (NFRA; Taylor & Thorne, 2013). Also in keeping with SPJ principles, this tool is theory driven (Hart et al., 2011). It works within the functional analysis framework (Jackson, 1994; Jackson et al., 1987), which acts as a systematic guide for gathering risk-relevant information on firesetting recidivism. However, unlike the SAFARI, the NFRA was not designed to augment an existing risk assessment tool (e.g., HCR-20). It was designed with its own list of factors derived from the theory and firesetting recidivism literature. Thus, the NFRA is based on a multi-factor explanation of firesetting behaviour that captures background and childhood factors, static and dynamic risk factors, proximal triggers, and offence-specific details. Taken together, this information is developed into a clinical formulation that conceptualises an individual's risk of reoffending, treatment targets (including prioritisation), intervention plan, and responsivity issues, as well as opportunities for ongoing updates along the treatment pathway.

Modelling evidence-based tools such as the HCR-20, Taylor and Thorne (2005) developed the NFRA to structure the collation of risk-relevant information along historical and clinical factors empirically linked to firesetting. In one of its earlier iterations, the NFRA guided clinicians to rate five historical factors and six clinical factors (Taylor & Thorne, 2013). However, evolving with the research developments (see Taylor & Thorne, 2019), the NFRA is now structured as follows:

- Historical items: (1) incidents of childhood firesetting, (2) previous incidents of firesetting as an adult, (3) previous incidents of targeted firesetting, (4) misuse of emergency services, (5) previous self-harm or suicidal gestures, (6) absence of interpersonal violence, (7) personality disorder, (8) incidents indicative of a revenge motive, (9) victim of child abuse/neglect, and (10) substance use problems.
- Clinical items: (1) recent depression and/or stress, (2) high levels of anger, (3) social ineffectiveness, (4) impulsivity, (5) current or recent signs of major mental illness, (6) low social attention or feeling not "listened to", (7) low self-esteem, (8) fascination or attraction to fires or fire-related paraphernalia, (9) impoverished social support networks, (10) male gender.

The risk-relevant information is gathered from a range of sources (i.e., the client, client records, psychometric measures, staff observations) using a variety of methods (e.g., client interview, self-report questionnaires, multi-disciplinary team consultations, case file review). Further, Taylor et al. (2004) designed the Pathological Firesetters Interview (PFSI) to gather as much information from the client via semi-structured interview on socio-demographic characteristics and offending history (general and fire specific), historical situational factors (e.g., family background, educational attainment, adverse childhood experiences), historical dispositional factors (e.g., mental health diagnoses, intellectual disabilities and physical disabilities), proximal factors (e.g., immediate changes in mental health, interpersonal conflict, drug or alcohol misuse), and firesetting incident characteristics (i.e., motivations, alone or with others, affective response during/after).

The details gathered from the interview are augmented by additional sources of information aimed at validating client accounts and filling in gaps of knowledge. Given that people who set fires also hold offence-specific attitudes and beliefs, Taylor and Thorne (2013, 2019) recommend fire-specific questionnaires that can be used to evidence the presence of these attitudes in the risk assessment. The Fire Setting Assessment Schedule (FSAS) and Fire Interest Rating Scale (FIRS) were both developed by Murphy and Clare (1996) for use with people with an intellectual disability. They assess the feelings and cognitions that reinforce firesetting behaviour (e.g., "I started fires because I felt angry with people"; FSAS) and endorse firesetting situations (e.g., "Watching people run from a fire"; FIRS). Taylor and Thorne (2013, 2019) also recommend the Fire Assessment Scale (FAS; Muckley, 1997) to capture clients' attitudes towards firesetting beliefs and behaviours (e.g., "People often set fires when they are angry").[1]

In addition to the fire-specific factors outlined so far, it is recognised that people who set fires have other clinical factors noted in the literature as commonly associated with firesetting behaviour. Taylor and Thorne (2013, 2019) recommend assessing anger management and regulation (Novaco Anger Scale; Novaco, 2003), depression (Beck Depression Inventory-Short Form; Beck & Beck, 1972), and self-esteem (Culture-Free Self-Esteem Inventory, 2nd Edition; Battle, 1992).

This approach to risk assessment is both theory-driven and action-oriented, which allows for effective clinical formulation (Hart et al., 2011). It also benefits from evidenced, but not evaluated, development and implementation in forensic settings with a clinical population. However, there are limitations to its broader utility. For example, the design and protocol are intended for individuals with intellectual disabilities (Taylor & Thorne, 2019), which accounts for a subset of the firesetting population. It is also worth noting there are theoretical gaps in the functional analytic paradigm (see Chapter 3 for more detailed discussion). For example, there are limitations in the scope of distal factors (e.g., only very specific negative childhood experiences are incorporated), dynamic risk factors (e.g., fire-related scripts are neglected), and proximal factors (e.g., thoughts and feelings that trigger and/or reinforce firesetting behaviour) that would aid clinical formulation. Also, functional analysis theory takes more of a deficits-based approach, with little guidance on extracting the protective factors for (1) added explanatory power in the clinical formulation and (2) promoting desistance through a positive, strengths-based treatment plan. Omissions, such as the ones highlighted here, are surprising given that the NFRA has been very recently updated (Taylor & Thorne, 2019). Finally, and most important, the NFRA, like other firesetting risk assessment tools, has not been rigorously evaluated on its effectiveness to predict and attenuate risk.

Risk Assessment Using the Multi-Trajectory Theory of Adult Firesetting (M-TTAF)

In light of the approaches discussed thus far, one approach that appears to address several of the limitations discussed is to adopt the SPJ (*third generation*) method of risk assessment, guided by the M-TTAF (see Chapter 3 for detailed overview of the theory). This approach to risk assessment is currently the most up-to-date protocol that accounts for a wider range of firesetting variables (e.g., childhood experiences, motivations, triggers, and protective factors).

When adopting this approach, there are three key stages that culminate in a risk assessment report that is evidence-based and accessible to a multi-disciplinary clinical team. First, the M-TTAF provides a framework for the information gathering process by outlining the types of factors that have been found to be associated to firesetting behaviour. This process involves collating the information from a range of sources (i.e., clinical interview, file review, multi-disciplinary team consultations, validated psychometric tools). The presence or absence of relevant factors must then be presented in a narrative as part of the second stage: clinical formulation. The M-TTAF can inform this stage because it is an etiological theory that outlines how the factors interact with each other to produce the firesetting behaviour. The final and most crucial stage is the preparation of risk scenarios and a risk management plan. The outcome of this stage is a conceptualisation of the circumstances under which the reoffending will occur again and the practical steps that can be taken to attenuate the likelihood of reoffending.

Information-Gathering Process

The M-TTAF guides the process of identifying relevant information for the following categories: (1) historical factors, (2) clinical factors, (3), reinforcing factors, and (4) protective factors.

Historical factors. The *developmental context* is key to any clinical formulation explaining how and why clinical problems may have emerged. For example, it can signpost why particular offence-supportive attitudes and beliefs have emerged (Hart et al., 2011) and shed light on how ingrained such beliefs are. To illustrate, someone who developed offence-supportive attitudes in early childhood from their familial context will require higher intensity treatment to shift these beliefs compared with someone who developed those attitudes at an older age. Therefore, historical factors are integral to effective decision-making regarding risk management planning.

The M-TTAF extends beyond adverse childhood experiences described in previous tools to also include caregiver environment, social, and cultural factors that inform learning opportunities as well as biological or dispositional factors that inform how an individual interacts with their environment throughout stages of development. The aim of investigating the developmental context is usually two-fold: (1) to establish a history of firesetting behaviour and (2) to contextualise the development of dispositional characteristics (e.g., maladaptive coping, poor self regulation) that explain why an individual responds to proximal triggers with offending behaviour. Crucially, the M-TTAF is the only theoretical framework to account for the development of scripts or schemas. Scripts are cognitive rules that influence how we interpret and evaluate cues from internal (e.g., physiological arousal) and external (e.g., interpersonal interactions) stimuli (Tomkins, 1991). Often, they develop from childhood experiences, hence the importance of gathering this information when conducting risk assessment. Examples of relevant experiences may include early memories of watching fire events (e.g., bonfires) and recalling associated sensory stimulation, admiration of others who set fires (e.g., a family member), and inconsistent or problematic caregiver responses to own firesetting behaviour. These childhood experiences contextualise the development of clinical factors implicated in the firesetting behaviour during adulthood.

Clinical factors. The *developmental context* highlights features and mechanisms that give rise to dispositional and socio-cognitive factors that facilitate offending behaviour. The M-TTAF conceptualises these factors as *psychological vulnerabilities or strengths* that when "triggered" become *critical risk factors*—i.e., prompting the firesetting behaviour. These factors are an inappropriate interest in fire and fire paraphernalia, inappropriate scripts about fire (e.g., fire is the best way to destroy evidence; Butler & Gannon, 2015, 2021), supportive attitudes and beliefs about firesetting as well as antisocial behaviour, anger management and regulation, problem solving, and communication problems. To augment information gathering from clinical interview, there are several validated psychometric instruments that can be used (Table 4.1).

In addition to assessing the presence or absence of psychological vulnerabilities, clinical consideration is needed regarding the role of mental health. The M-TTAF presents mental health not as a key predictor but rather a moderator that can either exacerbate or attenuate the impact proximal factors have on psychological vulnerabilities. Therefore, when articulating the function of mental health in a clinical formulation (to be described further below), it is often the impact on the individual's capacity in relation to effective decision-making and coping that is particularly noteworthy.

Reinforcing factors. An integral part of risk assessment—in addition to explaining how and why the offending behaviour occurred in the first place—is explaining how and

Table 4.1 Validated psychometric tools to evaluate presence of psychological vulnerabilities.

Psychological Vulnerability	Psychometric Tool
Identification with fire Serious or pathological fire Interest Fire safety Fire interest Inappropriate fire scripts	• Four Factor Fire Scales (Ó Ciardha et al., 2015c) • Firesetting Questionnaire (Gannon et al., in preparation)
Offence-supportive attitudes: general Fire normalisation	• The Measure of Criminal Attitudes and Associates—Part B (Kroner & Mills, 2002; Mills & Kroner, 2001) • Firesetting Questionnaire—Firesetting as Normal Subscale (Gannon et al., in preparation)
Self/emotional regulation	• Novaco Anger Scale and Provocation Inventory (Novaco, 2003) • Barratt Impulsiveness Scale (Patton et al., 1995) • Coping Strategies Inventory—Short Form (Addison et al., 2007)
Social functioning issues	• Attachment Style Questionnaire (Feeney et al., 1994)
Self-concept	• The Culture-Free Self-Esteem Inventory—General (Battle, 1992) • The Nowicki-Strickland Locus of Control (Nowicki, 1976)

why someone might want to engage in the offending behaviour *again*. The M-TTAF explains the maintenance of firesetting behaviour through cognitive and affective processes that reinforce the predisposing attitudes and beliefs. This can take the form of positive affective responses (i.e., raise in mood), sensory stimulation, feelings of empowerment, and/or instrumental gains (e.g., financial reward). Most important is consideration of the valence of the reinforcement. For example, if the reinforcement effect is rooted in positive affect and associated cognition, this could result in an individual viewing their behaviour as a method of effective goal pursuit. If, on the other hand, the reinforcement effect is rooted in negative affect and cognition, this could reinforce the psychological vulnerabilities by upholding negative world views and associated schemas. The most valuable sources of information on reinforcing factors are likely to be the clinical interview (i.e., eliciting an individual's thoughts and feelings in response to the firesetting offence) and case file information (e.g., insurance claims).

Protective factors. A clinical risk formulation is most helpful to treatment planning if it also articulates protective factors that can be reinforced and augmented to support desistance. Although the firesetting literature on protective factors is impoverished, there are adjacent literatures that can guide the information-gathering phase. Protective factors, in the wider forensic psychological literature, are typically clustered into five domains: internal resilience factors (e.g., coping strategies), treatment-related factors (e.g., treatment compliance), social factors (e.g., prosocial peers), environmental factors (e.g., residential accommodation), and community reintegration factors (e.g., employment opportunities; de Vries Robbé & Willis, 2017). The presence of any combination of the factors from these domains is likely to serve as a buffer when triggers or proximal factors arise. Unlike its predecessors, the M-TTAF also captures both internal and external factors that facilitate firesetting desistance. Individuals who set fires may experience an identity change that can be internally motivated from their own cognitive processing of the event and consequences, such as internalising responsibility and re-appraisals of cost and benefit. This identity change can also be facilitated by psychological interventions that result in problem-solving and communication skills development and/or the formation of prosocial goals with associated prosocial attitudes. Finally, the M-TTAF explicates the importance of external influences such as social support (e.g., family support, new intimate partner) and other environmental or situational changes (e.g., new employment, stable housing).

Clinical Formulation

The presence or absence of the factors outlined in this chapter only tell a part of a person's story. To fully understand how and why a person has offended, a risk assessment must also include a clinical formulation (i.e., a narrative of how the factors interacted and contributed to the index and or previous firesetting behaviour). The key objectives of clinical formulation are to (1) gather and organise the information needed to understand why and how the offending occurred, (2) involve the client (where ever possible) so that the process is collaborative, (3) "connect the dots" (i.e., present the inter-relationships between factors), (4) offer insights as to likely intervention opportunities, and (5) communicate risk-relevant information including which aspects to prioritise clinically (Logan, 2014). The outcome of an effective clinical formulation is a narrative that is accessible by a multi-disciplinary team so all aspects of the individual (e.g., education, family support, psychological wellbeing) can be addressed.

As mentioned previously, the M-TTAF is an etiological theory that presents how the factors interact. As such, it can be used to guide the generation of a clinical formulation. For example, historical factors should be framed in how they give rise to current, clinical factors (e.g., criminogenic needs such as fire-related scripts). The clinical factors need to be contextualised amongst proximal factors and triggers in order to highlight which factors need to be prioritised in treatment. Crucially, there needs to be an explanation of how this behaviour is reinforced. That is, why would the individual want to set fires in the future? But ultimately, the clinical formulation must also offer clinicians with target areas to build upon so the individual is motivated to engage (i.e., protective factors). The M-TTAF offers a template for generating the clinical formulation in risk assessment.

Risk scenarios and risk management plan. In addition to providing the framework for knitting together a clinical formulation, the M-TTAF can be used as a comprehensive storyboard for producing the likely scenarios that could result in the individual's setting future fires. The nature of risk is dynamic. Risk of reoffending can increase or decrease, and the main aim of risk scenarios is to offer narrative examples of "possible futures" and the conditions or parameters therein (Douglas et al., 2013b). In other words, what could happen in the future in light of this individual's clinical formulation? Risk scenarios must seem plausible and capture the risk factors identified in the previous steps of the risk assessment. It is also important for the scenarios to highlight contextual or environmental influences. For example, clinical concerns may vary depending upon where the individual resides (i.e., hospital or prison versus community), which also vary in levels of supervision and monitoring. The HCR-20 Version 3 guidance on writing risk scenarios offers a useful framework on how to capture relevant yet varied scenarios to inform risk management plans (Douglas et al., 2013). Clinicians are advised to write as many scenarios that are deemed helpful in devising a risk management plan, but there are four types that maximise their utility.

First, it is helpful to begin with a scenario similar to the reference or index offence (i.e., "repeat" scenario). If, for example, the clinical formulation included *psychological vulnerabilities* such as poor or maladaptive coping strategies and *proximal factors* such as a life event (e.g., bereavement) as precursors to the firesetting incident, a potential risk scenario would include the possibility of having to cope with another significant life event. The scenario would outline a similar context (e.g., living alone in the community), with similar levels of support and/or supervision. This scenario makes the assumption that not much has changed in the individual's life, which makes them equally vulnerable and prone to firesetting behaviour to cope. This is a useful starting point given that the index offence has likely resulted in their current placement for assessment.

An equally informative scenario is one that presents an "optimistic" possible future. The aim of this scenario is to outline the circumstances where risk of reoffending decreases. Building on the previous scenario, for example, an optimistic scenario might describe an individual who has developed effective coping strategies (e.g., communication with professionals, cognitive techniques to manage negative emotions) that promote resilience. The scenario could also describe plausible, prosocial life circumstances such as employment and/or recreational activities that counter their past experiences of social isolation. This scenario raises awareness to the clinical team on possible treatment targets, while highlighting the potential protective factors to be harnessed.

It is also important to consider a "worst case" scenario. This is the type of scenario when the offending escalates with greater potential for increased damage or harm (e.g., life-threatening harm). In this type of scenario, it is key to conceptualise what would happen if the individual's psychological vulnerabilities have become more extreme resulting in the belief that more drastic measures are needed. For example, if an individual experiences additional life events (e.g., further bereavements, relationship breakdown), they might adopt the thinking style that "life is no longer worth living." The firesetting that was previously a form of help-seeking behaviour could escalate to attempted suicide.

The final scenario type worth conceptualising is one that involves a "twist." This type of scenario is intended to capture ways in which the offending behaviour could evolve. A useful strategy in developing "twist" scenarios is considering how the environment influences the offending behaviour. For example, an individual who sets fire in the community is more likely than someone in custody to have access to a variety of materials (e.g., accelerants, combustible materials) and opportunities (e.g., no supervision). Once in custody, given the nature of the offending, this individual would no longer have this unsupervised access. As a twist scenario, it could be helpful to explore alternative forms of satiating an inappropriate fire interest (if highlighted in the clinical formulation), such as generating sparks from electrical appliances and/or sockets. The aim of this type of scenario is to "think outside the box" to put in place a risk management plan that considers how offending behaviour can evolve as circumstances change.

These scenarios facilitate the development of an individualised risk management plan that is designed to address the concerns raised in the scenarios. These scenarios aid the prioritisation of risk and protective factors when intervention planning. If coping with significant life events is viewed as high priority, then the risk management plan will involve intervention work to develop helpful coping strategies to manage negative affective responses to life events. The plan would also alert staff to update their supervision strategies if new life events arise. Similarly, if conflict resolution is an area for concern, then the risk management plan will involve intervention work on anger regulation and possibly communication skills. Last, the risk management plan is best developed by a multi-disciplinary team to account for the range of risk and protective factors, which do not all require psychological intervention.

Conclusions, Ways of Working, and Future Directions

General risk assessment processes have evolved over the past few decades as a result of sustained research. Yet the firesetting literature, although gaining traction, is still in its infancy. As a result, risk assessments for firesetting are limited in number and remain unvalidated. Nonetheless, the aim of this chapter is to offer best practice strategies that are action-oriented and theory-driven.

Firesetting risk assessment has clinical and practical implications for many layers of the criminal justice system. Actuarial (*second-generation*) tools give us insight into the probability someone will reoffend. For individuals with limited engagement with psychological services, this method offers a cost-effective triage approach to inform decision-making on placement (e.g., community versus custody) and intervention intensity.

The SPJ (*third-generation*) approach, however, addresses all three questions that opened this chapter. This method produces a clinical risk formulation that (1) explains how the offence occurred; (2) evaluates the likelihood, given current circumstances, the offence will happen again; and (3) outlines practical steps to attenuate risk (i.e., the risk management plan). As discussed in Chapter 3, the M-TTAF is the most up-to-date theoretical framework based on the latest research developments. As such, the historical, clinical, reinforcing, and protective factors described consist of both static risk factors with predictive validity and dynamic (criminogenic) risk factors that offer targets for treatment. The M-TTAF can act also as a template for developing clinical formulations and risk planning scenarios. These are essential to risk management plans that are effective. However, similar to other approaches discussed in this chapter, the M-TTAF as an aide to the SPJ method of risk assessment has neither been evaluated nor validated. It does, however, knit together the two leading theoretical models on firesetting behaviour and clinical risk assessment and formulation. With this in mind, it is the role of the clinician to continue to synchronise practice with the latest developments in theory and research.

Regardless of the approach taken, transparency being paramount, the following core principles are recommended when preparing a risk assessment report:

- Highlight the limited state of the literature and specifically note the lack of standardised tools;
- Clearly specify (and signpost) the theory and research evidence used to guide your risk assessment; and
- Given the heterogeneity of this type of offending behaviour, prepare an individualised clinical risk formulation and risk management plan to capture nuanced differences.

As more clinicians adopt fire-specific approaches to risk assessment, more opportunities for evaluation of implementation and validation of predictive strength emerge. The heterogeneity of firesetting behaviour requires an individualised approach because it highlights challenges that require specific attention from researchers and clinicians alike. For example, research to validate risk assessment protocols needs to consider institutional settings (prison versus hospital). Also, risk assessments need to be sensitive to the gender differences inherent in offending behaviour generally and evidenced in firesetting specifically (Alleyne et al., 2016). As the firesetting literature grows, we hope that researchers and professionals will turn their attentions towards developing validated and theoretically informed risk assessments.

Note

1 These measures are presented here for the purposes of outlining the NFRA's recommended approach. Latest developments on fire-specific measures are outside the scope of this chapter. Chapter 6 provides detailed discussion of validated measures.

5

Un-apprehended Deliberate Firesetting: Can We Intervene?

The detection and clearance rates for deliberate fires are very low (see Chapter 1). For example, in England and Wales between 2015 and 2016, there were 21,961 cases of arson recorded by the police and only 1,242 successful prosecutions, representing a 5.7% clearance rate (Arson Prevention Forum, 2017). In the US, the Federal Bureau of Investigation (FBI) Uniform Crime Reporting Statistics illustrate a 21.7% clearance rate (by arrest) for known arson offences in 2017 (FBI, 2018a). Similarly, in Canada, only 16% of reported arson offences were cleared "by charge or otherwise" in 2018 (Statistics Canada, 2019). These figures indicate that a large proportion of individuals responsible for deliberate fires go un-apprehended by authorities. The number of individuals who remain un-apprehended for deliberate firesetting presents a serious issue for agencies and policy makers involved in the prevention and reduction of intentional fires in terms of knowing how many people are responsible for these incidents, identifying potential risk factors for this behaviour, and knowing where and how to target resources.

In this chapter, recent research examining deliberate firesetting in the general population will be presented. In particular, we will describe the key characteristics, motivations, psychopathological, psychological, and behavioural features of community individuals who self-report deliberate firesetting. Comparisons will also be made between this group and individuals whose firesetting has been detected by services or criminal justice authorities. The chapter will then consider how the existing literature regarding those who have set fires and have not been apprehended can be applied practically by allied disciplines to inform prevention and intervention strategies to reduce this behaviour. Throughout this chapter, the term "un-apprehended" is used to refer to individuals who self-report having deliberately set a fire but never having been caught for this (i.e., they have not been identified by authorities for setting a fire nor have they ever been formally recorded for firesetting in official figures). In line with this, the term "apprehended" will be used to refer to research involving individuals who are formally known for having set fires.

Prevalence

Relatively few studies have examined the prevalence and characteristics of adults in the community who self-report setting fires. The first research in this area utilised data from Wave 1 of the National Epidemiologic Survey on Alcohol and Related Conditions in the US

Adult Deliberate Firesetting: Theory, Assessment, and Treatment, First Edition. Theresa A. Gannon, Nichola Tyler, Caoilte Ó Ciardha and Emma Alleyne.
© 2022 John Wiley & Sons Ltd. Published 2022 by John Wiley & Sons Ltd.

(NESARC; Blanco et al., 2010; Vaughn et al., 2010). The Wave 1 NESARC represents a cross-sectional nationally representative survey of 43,093 non-institutionalised adults in the US. Data were collected on participants' backgrounds, alcohol use, and comorbid health conditions (e.g., demographics, psychopathology, behavioural factors, substance use, and medical conditions) using face-to-face interviews conducted by trained Census workers. Within the survey interview module on antisocial personality disorder, a single question asked about participants' history of firesetting: "In your entire life did you ever start a fire on purpose to destroy someone else's property or just to see it burn?" This was then categorised as occurring before or after 15 years of age. Using this screening question, the lifetime prevalence of firesetting in the US community population was calculated as 1.0% to 1.13% (Blanco et al., 2010; Vaughn et al., 2010)—1.7% in men and 0.4% in women (Hoertel et al., 2011). Just over 60% of participants reported that their firesetting occurred before the age of 15 years; however, just under 40% reported that they had set fires after 15 years of age (Blanco et al., 2010).

Whilst the NESARC represents the first research to specifically examine the prevalence of self-reported firesetting in the adult general population, some methodological issues may have impacted the prevalence rates reported. First, the single question used to identify those who had engaged in firesetting was very vague. It is therefore possible that participants who had set socially or culturally sanctioned fires (e.g., campfires, bonfires, stubble burning) or who engaged in child fire play or experimentation with fire may have endorsed this item (Dickens & Sugarman, 2012; Gannon & Barrowcliffe, 2012). Second, the question only focused on fires set to "destroy someone else's property or just to see it burn," which does not reflect the range of targets or motivations identified in the existing literature as being associated with deliberate firesetting (e.g., setting fire to hurt oneself or another). Third, interviews for the NESARC were conducted face to face; consequently, social desirability or fear of reprisal may have inhibited participants' responses (Dickens & Sugarman, 2012; Gannon & Barrowcliffe, 2012). Finally, as only a single question was used to assess firesetting, it is unclear if any of the respondents had ever been formally charged for this behaviour or how prolific firesetting was for those who responded affirmatively (Barrowcliffe & Gannon, 2015). These methodological limitations mean that the prevalence of firesetting detected in the NESARC likely under-represents the true occurrence of this behaviour in the general population.

Gannon and Barrowcliffe attempted to address some of these issues in their series of UK community studies (Barrowcliffe, 2017; Barrowcliffe & Gannon, 2015, 2016; Gannon & Barrowcliffe, 2012). To address the influence of social desirability, Gannon and Barrowcliffe invited participants to complete an anonymous survey which asked them to self-report if they had ever set a deliberate fire over the age of 10 years. To improve upon the methodological and specificity issues associated with the NESARC question, Gannon and Barrowcliffe provided more detailed operational definitions of both deliberate firesetting (e.g., to "annoy other people, to relieve boredom, to create excitement, for insurance purposes, as a result of peer pressure, or to get rid of evidence") and non-problematic or unintentional firesetting (e.g., "for organized events such as bonfires, fires started accidentally"). Individuals who indicated they had engaged in acts of deliberate firesetting (as defined earlier) were then asked to provide further information about this (e.g., number of fires started, age when they set the fire(s), and motivation for setting the fire(s)). In their first study, Gannon and Barrowcliffe (2012) surveyed 168 university students and found that 11% ($n = 18$) reported having set an intentional fire. Notably, only 1.3% ($n = 2$) reported having set fires during adulthood. Although Gannon and Barrowcliffe (2012) refined and improved upon the methodology used in the NESARC study, their university student sample—which was predominantly female—limited the conclusions that could be drawn about the prevalence of deliberate firesetting in the wider community.

To address these limitations, Barrowcliffe and Gannon (2015) surveyed adult community participants, recruited via a postal survey that was hand delivered to 10% of houses in an area with a high number of recorded deliberate fires, within one district of the UK ($n = 158$). In this study, a similar proportion of participants reported having set a deliberate fire (11.5%; $n = 18$). Furthermore, the majority (>80%) of participants reported that they had set multiple fires, and just over a third (38.9%; $n = 7$) reported that they had set their most recent deliberate fire as an adult. In their third study, Barrowcliffe and Gannon (2016) recruited a larger sample of community participants using social media and snowballing techniques ($n = 225$). In this study, 17.78% ($n = 40$) of participants self-reported having set a deliberate fire since the age of 10 years, of these 62.5% ($n = 25$) reported setting more than one deliberate fire, and 15% ($n = 6$) reported having set a deliberate fire as an adult. In a fourth study, Barrowcliffe et al. (2022) narrowed the focus and examined self-reported firesetting in community adults age 18 to 23 years. The concentration on this group was in response to findings from the previous studies which indicated that the majority of participants began lighting fires in adolescence. Thus, there were concerns about potential memory effects for older participants who were being asked to recall behaviours that may have occurred many years before. Participants were recruited using the crowdsourcing platform Prolific Academic ($n = 240$). Twenty-five percent of participants ($n = 60$) reported having set a fire since the age of 10 years, with 55% ($n = 33$) of this group reporting having set multiple fires. For those who reported setting a fire(s), the average age of last fire set was 16 years; however, 35% ($n = 21$) reported that they continued to light fires after the age of 18 years.

Barrowcliffe and Gannon's work indicate that the true prevalence of intentional firesetting in the general population is likely to be higher than that detected in the NESARC studies. In fact, the pooled prevalence across Gannon and Barrowcliffe's three earliest studies suggests that approximately 14% of the general population self-report having deliberately set a fire after the age of 10 years. These studies have also developed methodologies that have enabled us, for the first time, to estimate the number of people responsible for deliberate firesetting, something which incident and clearance data are unable to account for.

Characteristics and Psychological Features

Until recently, knowledge about the characteristics, clinical features, and motivations of individuals who set deliberate fires had been restricted to research with individuals who have come to the attention of authorities for their firesetting (e.g., criminal justice and mental health services), with a distinct focus on those convicted of arson offences (Dickens & Sugarman, 2012). However, research utilising data from the NESARC in the US (e.g.,

Blanco et al., 2010; Hoertel et al., 2011; Vaughn et al., 2010) as well as that systematically investigating un-apprehended firesetting in UK community samples (e.g., Barrowcliffe, 2017; Barrowcliffe & Gannon, 2015, 2016; Barrowcliffe et al., 2019, in press; Gannon & Barrowcliffe, 2012), has advanced current knowledge of the characteristics, psychopathology, motivations, psychological features, and crime scene behaviours of un-apprehended firesetting individuals. To develop effective prevention strategies, it is critical that we understand any similarities and differences between those who are identified for deliberate firesetting and those who are not. In this section, recent research on the characteristics of un-apprehended firesetting individuals will be discussed and comparisons made with the apprehended firesetting literature.

Gender

Research with those apprehended for firesetting suggests this to be a predominantly male perpetrated crime, with gender ratios ranging from approximately 3:1 male to female to 6:1 male to female (Anwar et al., 2011; Ducat et al., 2017; Enayati et al., 2008; see Chapter 2). In the nationally representative NESARC studies, for every woman reporting deliberate firesetting there were almost five men (Blanco et al., 2010; Hoertel et al., 2011; Vaughn et al., 2010). In contrast, the small sample research conducted in the UK by Barrowcliffe and Gannon suggests a much closer gender ratio. For example, Barrowcliffe and Gannon (2015) reported that 61.1% of those who self-reported having set a fire were male, and 38.9% were female, a ratio of 1.5:1 male to female (see also Barrowcliffe & Gannon, 2016). Taken together, these findings suggest that females may be represented at a higher rate in un-apprehended firesetting samples.

Developmental Experiences

Adult individuals apprehended for firesetting tend to self-report the majority of their firesetting to have occurred in adulthood (Gannon et al., 2015). Similarly to non-firesetting individuals who have offended, they tend to be characterised by low socio-economic status, high levels of non-completion of compulsory schooling, and a history of unemployment or low skilled employment (see Gannon & Pina, 2010; Smith & Short, 1995). They also come from large and financially disadvantaged families, are likely to have experienced neglect or abuse (e.g., physical, sexual, or emotional abuse), and have a family member who has set fires (Gannon & Pina, 2010).

Research with un-apprehended adult firesetting samples suggests these individuals have set the majority of their fires during mid to late adolescence (Barrowcliffe, 2017; Barrowcliffe & Gannon, 2015, 2016; Gannon & Barrowcliffe, 2012). This group report themselves to be well educated (e.g., hold qualifications of high school level and above), to have a good personal and family income, and have a developmental history largely free from neglect and abuse. However, like apprehended individuals, they are likely to have a family member who has set fires (Barrowcliffe & Gannon, 2015, 2016; Blanco et al., 2010; Vaughn et al., 2010). These findings suggest that in comparison to apprehended firesetting individuals, those who remain un-apprehended for firesetting set the majority of their fires in adolescence and are academically able yet lack parental boundaries.

Finally, it is worth noting that factors relevant to the developmental context (i.e., genetics and neurobiological factors) have not been examined in relation to un-apprehended firesetting (see Chapter 2 for information on these factors in relation to apprehended firesetting).

Offending or Antisocial Behaviour

Research examining the offence histories of those apprehended for firesetting suggests this population have high rates of criminal convictions and are criminally versatile (Ducat et al., 2013a; Soothill et al., 2004). They also appear to engage in other antisocial behaviours (i.e., problematic behaviours that do not necessarily result in a criminal conviction). For example, a recent meta-analytic review comparing firesetting and non-firesetting youth identified that firesetting youth had significantly more extensive histories of antisocial and problematic behaviours (e.g., cruelty, aggression, assaultive behaviour, disruptive behaviour outburst, lying, inappropriate behaviour, oppositional behaviour, truancy, school behavioural problems) than non-firesetting youth (Perks et al., 2019).

The findings are less clear for un-apprehended firesetting adults. Analysis of the NESARC found a self-reported personal and family history of antisocial behaviour was significantly higher among individuals with a history of self-reported firesetting than those without this history (Blanco et al., 2010; Vaughn et al., 2010), a finding consistent across men and women (Hoertel et al., 2011). The most prevalent self-reported antisocial behaviours included doing something you could have been arrested for, cutting class without permission, staying out late at night, shoplifting, stealing from others, destroying others' property, and doing things that could easily hurt you or others (Blanco et al., 2010; Vaughn et al., 2010). Differences were observed in the prevalence of antisocial behaviours across men and women. For example, cutting class, getting three or more traffic tickets for reckless driving, having a driver's licence suspended, and using a weapon in a fight were significantly associated with firesetting in women but not in men, whereas hurting an animal on purpose, failing to pay off personal debts, and shoplifting were significantly associated with firesetting in men but not women (Hoertel et al., 2011). Although individuals who had set fires reported significantly higher levels of antisocial behaviour, criminal convictions were not captured as part of the NESARC. Thus, it is unclear if any of the participants had received a criminal conviction for their self-reported antisocial behaviours.

In comparison, Barrowcliffe and Gannon (2015, 2016) found no difference between firesetting and non-firesetting participants on self-reported history of school expulsion and criminal convictions. However, individuals who self-reported deliberate firesetting were significantly more likely than non-firesetting individuals to report having been suspended from school and scored significantly higher on measures of antisocial attitudes (Barrowcliffe & Gannon, 2016). A later study by Barrowcliffe et al. (2022) examined specific types of unconvicted antisocial behaviour in a sample of 18- to 23-year old UK participants and found that relative to non-firesetting individuals, those who reported a history of firesetting were significantly more likely to report having engaged in robbery, assault, illegal substance use, shop theft, vandalism, and frequent truanting from school and to have criminal associates.

Taken together, these findings suggest that similar to those apprehended for firesetting, un-apprehended individuals are criminally versatile, socialise with antisocial family members and peers, and have a lifetime history of engaging in antisocial behaviour. However, their lack of criminal convictions suggests that similar to their firesetting, this antisocial behaviour may often not receive attention by authorities.

Psychopathology

Individuals apprehended for firesetting are often reported to have high levels of psychopathological need and high levels of engagement with mental health services, with schizophrenia and personality disorders (borderline and antisocial types) identified as common psychiatric diagnoses in this population (Barnett & Spitzer, 1994; Ducat et al., 2013b; Gannon & Pina, 2010; Ó Ciardha et al., 2015a; Tyler & Gannon, 2012; see Chapter 2). Research examining un-apprehended firesetting individuals indicates that this group also experience difficulties with psychological well-being and mental health. In the NESARC Wave 1, lifetime prevalence of mental illness and current physical, social, and emotional, and mental health functioning were screened for using the Alcohol Use Disorder and Associated Disabilities Interview Schedule–DSM-IV (AUDADIS-IV; Grant et al., 1995) and the Short Form 12v2 (SF-12v2; Ware et al., 2002). Analysis of the NESARC Wave 1 data (Blanco et al., 2010; Vaughn et al., 2010) found that individuals who self-reported a lifetime history of deliberate firesetting were significantly more likely than non-firesetting individuals to meet the criteria for a lifetime history of at least one psychiatric disorder on the AUDADIS-IV and to report having sought treatment for mental health issues. The strongest associations were found between firesetting history and antisocial personality disorder, drug dependence, pathological gambling, and bipolar disorder. Regarding current well-being, individuals with a self-reported history of firesetting had significantly lower scores on the social, emotional, and mental health subscales of the SF-12v2.

Barrowcliffe and Gannon (2015, 2016) also asked participants about various indicators of mental health (e.g., history of suicide attempts, self-harm, history of mental illness). Similar to the NESARC studies, firesetting participants were significantly more likely than non-firesetting participants to report having a diagnosis of a mental illness or behavioural disorder and to have engaged in suicide attempts and self-harming behaviours. These findings suggest that similar to individuals who have been apprehended for firesetting, un-apprehended firesetting individuals are likely to have poorer mental health outcomes than those who do not set fires. However, patterns in psychopathology and the relationship between particular symptoms and firesetting behaviour in this group are still unclear.

Psychological Features

Apprehended firesetting individuals can be differentiated from non-firesetting individuals on several aspects of psychological functioning, including higher levels of interest in and association with fire (e.g., serious fire interest and identification with fire), normalisation of fire use and misuse, and cognitive experiences of anger and provocation to anger (Gannon et al., 2013; see Chapter 2). Apprehended individuals who have set fires also hold lower levels of self-esteem and fire safety awareness (Gannon et al., 2013). Like apprehended individuals, those who remain un-apprehended for their firesetting also report significantly higher levels of interest in and association with fire (including fire-supportive attitudes), anger, and provocation relative to their non-firesetting community counterparts (Barrowcliffe & Gannon, 2015, 2016; Barrowcliffe et al., 2019; Gannon & Barrowcliffe, 2012). They also report significantly higher levels of boredom proneness and antisocial attitudes (Barrowcliffe & Gannon, 2016). Barrowcliffe et al. (2022) asked un-apprehended firesetting individuals what they thought would have prevented them from setting fires. The most commonly reported preventative measures included increased impulse control (35%, $n = 21$), fire safety knowledge (13.3%, $n = 8$), parental supervision (10%, $n = 6$), and confidence to stand up to peers (10%, $n = 6$). However, it is not possible to draw comparisons with apprehended firesetting individuals on these preventative factors because research has not asked both groups these questions.

These findings suggest that un-apprehended individuals have similar difficulties to their apprehended counterparts with self and emotional regulation, interests and associations with fire, and antisocial attitudes, However, boredom proneness appears to be a factor that is relatively distinctive amongst un-apprehended firesetting individuals. To determine whether this is a factor that significantly distinguishes between these two groups, discriminant studies that compare apprehended and un-apprehended firesetting samples are needed.

Motivation

A large body of research exists that has examined motivations for firesetting amongst apprehended or identified individuals. Common motivators identified in the literature include revenge (Koson & Dvoskin, 1982; Lewis & Yarnell, 1951; Prins, 1994; Rix, 1994), excitement (Bradford, 1982; Inciardi, 1970), cry for help or communication (Geller, 1992), protection (Tyler et al., 2014), self-injury or suicide (Dickens et al., 2007; Tyler et al., 2014), crime concealment (Prins, 1994), and vandalism (Inciardi, 1970; Rix, 1994). In comparison, very little research has examined motivators for firesetting in un-apprehended individuals. In the only two studies to examine this, Barrowcliffe and Gannon (2015, 2016) asked UK community participants about their self-reported motivations for their firesetting. Across the two studies, "curiosity or experimenting with fire" was the most commonly reported motive followed by "to create fun/excitement or alleviate boredom" and "love fire." Other less commonly reported motives included "dared or pranked" and "vandalism."

When comparing the motivators reported for apprehended and un-apprehended firesetting individuals, some observable differences can be seen. For example, motives identified in the apprehended literature predominantly reflect antisocial attitudes or behaviour (e.g., crime concealment, revenge, and vandalism) or issues associated with emotional expression and communication (e.g., revenge, cry for help or communication, protection, self-injury or suicide). In contrast, motivators identified in un-apprehended firesetting individuals predominantly reflect self-regulation issues (e.g., thrill seeking and boredom) and an interest in fire. These differences may also reflect why some individuals end up in custody or in the care of mental health services for firesetting behaviour and others do not. For example, if firesetting is part of an array of antisocial behaviour or directed towards a person (self or another), individuals may be more likely to come to the attention of authorities than those setting a fire out of curiosity or experimentation.

Fire Scene Behaviours

A distinct body of work exists examining the crime scene behaviours of individuals who have set fires. However, most of this research utilises police data of solved arson cases, with little research examining the fire scene behaviours of un-apprehended firesetting individuals. Apprehended firesetting individuals are reported to set fires alone and relatively close to home, with average reported distances ranging from less than 100 metres to 6.63 kilometres, dependent on the population, country, and whether the fire was emotionally or instrumentally motivated (Edwards & Grace, 2006; Fritzon, 2001; Fritzon et al., 2014; Wachi et al., 2007). In addition, intoxication at the time of the firesetting is common, and accelerant is frequently reported to be used (Lindberg et al., 2005; Ritchie & Huff, 1999). Common targets include institutions, public buildings, residences (own and others), vehicles, and commercial property (Canter & Fritzon, 1998; Fritzon et al., 2014; Ritchie & Huff, 1999; Rix, 1994), and accelerant use is relatively common (Ritchie & Huff, 1999).

Barrowcliffe and Gannon (2015, 2016) asked un-apprehended firesetting participants a series of forced choice questions about their fire scene behaviours, including their modus operandi (e.g., ignition, distance from home), the target of their firesetting, and their post-firesetting responses (e.g., whether they extinguished the fire or not). Across their studies, Barrowcliffe and Gannon found that the vast majority of firesetting participants reported having set fires with one or more others (65%–90% of participants across studies) and were sober at the time of their firesetting. In addition, approximately two thirds reported setting fires within walking distance of their home (i.e., less than a mile away). The majority of participants (63%–80%) reported lighting a single ignition point, with the most common targets reported including the countryside (e.g., grass, shrubbery); paper, books, or newspapers; empty or derelict garages, sheds, beach huts, or outside bins; and flammable liquids or items. In addition, the majority of firesetting participants reported that they attempted to extinguish their fires.

Differences in fire scene characteristics between un-apprehended and apprehended firesetting individuals suggest that those who are detected are more likely to use accelerant and set fire to larger items of personal or public significance (e.g., public buildings, residences, commercial property), whereas those who go un-apprehended for their firesetting and predominantly report setting fire to smaller items (e.g., grass, paper, outside bins) or unused premises (e.g., derelict property). These differences also likely reflect risk of detection for firesetting. For example, fires set to smaller items and derelict properties are potentially more likely to go unnoticed, and those where accelerant are used may be larger and cause more noticeable damage. The varying distances travelled to the fire scene may also reflect an individual's ability to travel (e.g., access to transportation) and the motivations underpinning their firesetting. For example, as discussed previously, un-apprehended firesetting is reported to be motivated by curiosity, boredom, experimentation, and an interest in fire, motivators arguably driven by the need for immediate gratification. In contrast, apprehended firesetting individuals are more likely to be motivated by revenge, a cry for help, communication, and crime concealment, which may be more emotionally salient and more distally located.

Preventing Deliberate Firesetting

So far, this chapter has provided an overview of the emerging research on un-apprehended firesetting and compared it with the apprehended firesetting literature. Although still in its infancy, the emerging epidemiological research on those who remain un-apprehended for firesetting represents a significant advancement in the literature and provides much needed data on the prevalence and correlates of firesetting outside of those identified for this behaviour. Given that a perpetrator is not identified for the vast majority of deliberate fires, primary prevention initiatives are needed to reduce the incidence of this behaviour. Although we still know relatively little about those who remain un-apprehended for deliberate firesetting, the existing research in this area can provide us with some indicators on how and where to target prevention work and resources. In this section, an overview of existing prevention strategies for deliberate firesetting will be provided followed by an overview on how recent research examining un-apprehended firesetting can help inform the delivery of prevention initiatives.

Existing Prevention Strategies

Internationally, prevention and early intervention for firesetting are most commonly provided by fire and rescue services (Kolko et al., 2008; Muller & Stebbins, 2007; Palmer et al., 2005). Across North America, Australasia, and the UK, fire and rescue services deliver a range of initiatives to increase fire-safe behaviour and reduce the risk of deliberate firesetting. Some of these initiatives seek to improve the safety of property to reduce the risk of it being a target of firesetting (e.g., building design, surveillance, removal of fuel, security measures). Other strategies aim to change human behaviour such as diversion schemes (e.g., engagement programmes for at risk youth) and educational and informational programmes to empower communities with knowledge about fire safety and to deter people from misusing fire. Whilst environmental changes may remove opportunities for firesetting, behaviour change programmes seek to prevent people from engaging in the behaviour in the first place and/or modify problem behaviours early on. It is these interventions that the research on un-apprehended firesetting may be able to help inform and will be the focus of the rest of this chapter.

Behaviour change interventions for fire use predominantly comprise safety messaging in the form of parental education programmes (e.g., DVDs, leaflets, website resources, parent targeted home visits), national media campaigns, and fire safety education programmes. Many of these interventions aim to promote general fire safety awareness rather than reduce the risk of firesetting and are predominantly aimed at children and younger adolescents. For example, the majority of fire and rescue services offer fire safety education programmes in schools (Brown et al., 2013; Ogier, 2008) and for youth who set fires (see Kolko et al., 2008; Muller & Stebbins, 2007; Palmer et al., 2005). Consequently, the evidence base for fire prevention in youth is more developed than it is for older adolescents and adults. The small body of literature that has focused on behavioural change interventions in adults has predominantly focused on parents of young children and older adults.

Media campaigns have long been a popular channel for raising public awareness about the dangers of fire and delivering fire safety messages and are utilised in arson prevention strategies internationally (e.g., All Wales Joint Arson Group, 2019; Anderson, 2010; Brown et al., 2005). For example, during Arson Awareness Week, the US Fire Administration and Department of Homeland Security regularly publishes a range of outreach materials, media releases, and community resources to raise awareness of the dangers and consequences of deliberate firesetting, and many fire and rescue services have their own social media accounts, which they use to share information and safety messages. Media campaigns internationally tend to either focus on improving fire safety more generally (e.g., encouraging the use and testing of smoke alarms or having an escape plan) or reducing fire misuse more specifically. Whilst national media campaigns represent a potentially effective strategy for communicating the dangers of deliberate firesetting to a wide audience, there is a lack of published research on how effective these are in increasing safe fire practices.

Fire safety education programmes are one of the most commonly used prevention strategies to reduce fire misuse by educating people about the dangers of fire and encouraging safe behaviour around fire. Across many jurisdictions, fire safety education is delivered collaboratively by fire and rescue services and schools, with sessions often repeated at various stages of the curriculum (for an example, see Fire and Emergency New Zealand's Firewise programmes). However, fire safety education is a much less common approach for inducing behavioural change in adults, with those reported typically focusing on "at-risk," groups including parents of newborns (Hwang et al., 2006; Lehna et al., 2015a) and older adults (Lehna et al., 2015b, 2017; Walker et al., 1992). Research has reported mixed effects for adult fire safety education programmes with some studies observing short-term increases in fire safety knowledge (e.g., Lehna et al., 2015a, 2015b, 2017; Walker et al., 1992) and others finding little effect (e.g., Hwang et al., 2006). However, there is a lack of research examining the effectiveness of such education programmes with other adult groups (e.g., early to mid-adulthood). In addition, no research to date has examined if these interventions are effective in reducing the risk of the onset of firesetting or fire misuse.

Un-apprehended Deliberate Firesetting: Informing Prevention

Given the lack of evaluation of firesetting prevention initiatives, research examining the characteristics of those who go un-apprehended for this behaviour may provide some useful insight to help optimise existing strategies (e.g., potential intervention targets). In this section, how the emerging literature on un-apprehended firesetting may be used to inform existing primary prevention strategies for deliberate firesetting will be discussed.

When considering how to optimise firesetting prevention strategies, a key starting point is to identify the target audience and how best to capture them. As discussed earlier, recent research suggests that un-apprehended firesetting individuals are most likely to report setting fires during mid to late adolescence (Barrowcliffe & Gannon, 2015, 2016). They also appear to have high levels of educational attainment but regularly truant from school and have poor parental supervision (Barrowcliffe, 2017; Blanco et al., 2010; Vaughn et al., 2010). This suggests that whilst un-apprehended firesetting individuals are academically able, they are likely to be frequently absent from school and potentially lack parental guidance.

At present, the majority of primary prevention strategies for firesetting are aimed at young people, with fire safety messages directed at those younger than the age of 13 years and their caregivers (e.g., fire safety education). However, research with un-apprehended firesetting individuals suggests that it may be beneficial to develop prevention initiatives that are targeted at those older than 13 years of age. Further, due to poor school attendance, individuals engaged in un-apprehended firesetting are less likely to be captured by primary prevention initiatives delivered in schools. Whilst school-based fire safety sessions may be successful in conveying fire safety messages to a large proportion of the population, agencies tasked with fire prevention may also need to consider other mediums for communicating fire safety messages to young people. For example, delivering fire safety education through youth centres and sports societies or media outlets (including social media).

Although social media and television adverts are already being used by fire and rescue services, it is important to consider whether such media channels are effectively targeting young adults and whether the content of the message is having an impact. Lambie et al. (2018) asked New Zealand university students aged 17–24 years to rank potential mediums that could be used to promote safe fire behaviour amongst young adults. The top suggested mediums were Facebook, TV advertisements, fire service presentations, and YouTube. Further, participants were asked about how these messages could be delivered to improve safe fire behaviour in this age group. The most frequently suggested methods by participants included: increased or better fire safety education, campaigns or education that highlight the negative consequences of playing with fire, and campaigns designed or targeted specifically at young adults, suggesting that both the medium and the content of fire safety education campaigns are important to consider when trying to reach older youth.

Increasing parental supervision has been suggested by individuals who have gone un-apprehended for firesetting as a potential preventative strategy (Barrowcliffe et al., in press). Poor parental supervision has been found to be associated with engagement in offending behaviour more generally (Flanagan et al., 2019). Further, research suggests that this group are also likely to have poor psychological well-being (Barrowcliffe & Gannon, 2015, 2016; Blanco et al., 2010; Vaughn et al., 2010). It is therefore possible that individuals who have engaged in un-apprehended firesetting may be involved with other services (e.g., general practitioner, mental health services, social services). Whilst educating parents on safe fire practices may increase awareness of how to behave in the event of a fire, it may not directly address issues around supervision and reducing engagement in antisocial behaviour, including firesetting. Thus, making fire safety education available through other organisations (e.g., parenting programmes) may help prevent the onset of deliberate firesetting, through improving parental supervision as well as encouraging safe and appropriate fire behaviours.

As highlighted earlier, un-apprehended individuals who engage in firesetting are most likely to set fires out of curiosity or experimentation, to elicit excitement, to alleviate boredom, or because they have an interest in fire, and they often report setting fires with peers (Barrowcliffe & Gannon, 2015, 2016; Barrowcliffe et al., in press). Given these motivators, firesetting prevention initiatives may wish to consider strategies that focus on reducing the positive association or temptation surrounding fire in young people. In Western cultures, fire is often revered, and its use restricted, meaning that there are limited learning opportunities for young people to learn about the forms and functions of fire and safe fire behaviours (Gannon et al., 2012). Further, research suggests that a lack of knowledge about the dangers and consequences of fire misuse is associated with firesetting and unsafe fire behaviour in the general population (Barrowcliffe et al., in press; Lambie et al., 2018). It is important to consider ways in which services working to prevent deliberate firesetting may approach this. Traditional scare tactics are noted to be largely ineffective in encouraging attitudinal change towards fire and can in fact have adverse effects (e.g., increase problem behaviour or traumatise individuals; Lambie et al., 2015). The features of successful safety campaigns have been identified as those which challenge peer norms, use humour and positivity, and are tailored to the audience in question (e.g., age group; Lambie et al., 2015).

As discussed, the emerging research on un-apprehended deliberate firesetting offers useful information to help inform primary prevention strategies, providing data that can both guide and optimise existing initiatives. However, more research is needed to advance our understanding and knowledge of this little studied group including rigorous evaluation research to understand what preventative techniques are effective, with whom, when, and why.

Conclusions, Ways of Working, and Future Directions

Current prevention work for firesetting predominantly focuses on providing fire safety education to young people and their caregivers. Whilst offering fire safety education via different mediums holds some potential for reducing engagement in deliberate firesetting, this approach can arguably only target some of the known correlates associated with deliberate firesetting in un-apprehended individuals. Tyler et al. (2019a) have recently advocated for deliberate firesetting to be recognised and treated as a public health issue because of the significant impact this behaviour has on physical and psychological human well-being. Public health approaches adopt a population-based system-wide approach to preventing health issues (i.e., focusing on the whole population not just high-risk individuals; World Health Organization, 2011). Public health models are particularly appealing when considering how to tackle deliberate firesetting given so few perpetrators are apprehended or even identified. Current prevention and intervention strategies target only a proportion of those responsible for deliberately set fires (e.g., those younger than the age of 13 years and their caregivers, those formally identified as starting to misuse or detected for firesetting by services). A public health approach views firesetting as a preventable consequence of a range of social, psychological, economic, and environmental factors and utilises multi-agency working to target the root causes of firesetting, as opposed to focusing solely on the end outcome.

Developing a more detailed understanding of the demographic, psychological, and behavioural characteristics of those who go un-apprehended and/or remain un-apprehended for firesetting forms an important part of this research agenda, including discriminant studies that directly examine the similarities and differences between apprehended and un-apprehended firesetting individuals to identify key targets for intervening with these groups and to enable the design of tailored interventions. In addition, given the absence of research demonstrating the effectiveness of existing prevention initiatives in reducing the risk of onset of firesetting behaviour, applying a public health model could enable the development of best practice in firesetting prevention. For a public health model to be effectively applied to deliberate firesetting, multi-disciplinary collaboration is needed between policy makers, researchers, practitioners (e.g., criminal justice system, fire and rescue services, health, social care, and education), and the wider community. Thus, future research, policy, and practice could benefit from organising and aligning their agendas with that of a shared public health model to enable the systematic investigation and evaluation of the prevention of deliberate firesetting.

6

Assessment and Treatment for Apprehended Adults Who Have Set Deliberate Fires

Research suggests that a significant number of individuals residing in secure settings have a history of deliberate firesetting. Geller et al. (1992) reported that 17.8% of patients residing in a state hospital in the US had a lifetime history of intentional firesetting. Further, research from across the UK, Sweden, and Finland indicates that approximately 10%–14% of individuals admitted to forensic mental health services have a history of deliberate firesetting (Coid et al., 2001; Fazel & Grann, 2002; Hollin et al., 2013; Repo et al., 1997). The number of adults detained in prison for fire-related offences is unclear; however, between 2006 and 2011, the number of adults sentenced for arson offences in England and Wales ranged between 560 and 630 adults per year, 41% of whom were sentenced to immediate custody (Sentencing Council, 2018). Whilst these figures indicate a significant number of individuals are sentenced for arson offences each year, they likely under-represent the number of people currently incarcerated for fire-related offences. For example, they exclude those whose offending involves firesetting but who are convicted of offences other than arson (e.g., murder, criminal damage, taking without consent) as well as individuals who have set fires in custody but who have not received any formal conviction for this.

Given the number of apprehended individuals with a history of deliberate firesetting, it is critical that practitioners are able to appropriately assess and provide treatment for this behaviour to effectively manage firesetting risk (both within the secure environment and in the wider community) and to reduce reoffending (Tyler et al., 2019b). In this chapter, an overview of recent developments in assessment and treatment of adult firesetting is provided, including detailed descriptions of firesetting-specific measures and interventions and the evidence of their effectiveness. Whilst this chapter has a focus on assessment of adult firesetting, it does not specifically address risk assessment since this is covered in detail elsewhere (see Chapter 4).

Assessing Adult Firesetting

As discussed earlier in this volume, firesetting adults can be differentiated from non-firesetting adults on various psychological and background factors, including attitudes, associations, and interests in fire; anger cognition and provocation; self-esteem; locus of control orientation; engagement in firesetting in childhood; history of mental health issues and treatment; previous convictions for vandalism or property offences; and substance use (Alleyne et al., 2016; Ducat et al., 2013a, 2013b; Gannon et al., 2013; Tyler et al., 2015). Many of these factors are described within the latest theory of deliberate firesetting, the Multi-Trajectory Theory of Adult Firesetting (M-TTAF; Gannon et al., 2012; see also Chapter 3), as potential dynamic risk factors (or psychological vulnerabilities or strengths) that both facilitate and maintain firesetting (e.g., *inappropriate fire interest or fire scripts, offence-supportive attitudes, self/emotional regulation issues*, and *communication and relationship difficulties*). Some of these potential risk factors are similar to those identified for other offence types and therefore may be assessed using widely available measures. However, one particular area of dynamic risk that appears unique to firesetting is interests, attitudes, and associations with fire.

Having an interest or fascination with fire has consistently been found to be a key predictor for both the onset and repetition of firesetting behaviour (Kolko & Kazdin, 1992; McCarty & McMahon, 2005; Rice & Harris, 1996; Tyler et al., 2015). Given that fire-specific interests, associations, and attitudes appear to be important risk factors for deliberate firesetting, it is important to be able to accurately assess these factors to inform case formulation, treatment planning, and risk management. Whilst a variety of assessment tools are available to assess other factors associated with firesetting (e.g., *offence-supportive attitudes, self/emotional regulation*, and *communication and relationship difficulties*), only a small number have been developed specifically to assess fire-specific factors. In this section, an overview of tools designed to assess fire-specific factors in adults is provided and the strengths and weakness of each measure discussed. Five tools are considered: the Fire-setting Assessment Schedule (FAS; Murphy & Clare, 1996), Fire Setting Scale (FSS; Gannon & Barrowcliffe, 2012), Fire Proclivity Scale (FPS; Gannon & Barrowcliffe, 2012), Four Factor Fire Scale (FFFS; Ó Ciardha et al., 2015b, 2015c), and Firesetting Questionnaire (FQ; Gannon et al., in preparation).

Fire-setting Assessment Schedule (Murphy & Clare, 1996)

The FAS is a 32-item measure that was developed for use with adults with intellectual disabilities who have set fires to assess events, feelings, and cognitions preceding and following firesetting incidents. Eight constructs are assessed before and after firesetting: self-stimulation (e.g., "I felt that starting fires was the most exciting thing I could do"), anxiety (e.g., "I started fires because I felt worried or tense"), social attention (e.g., "I started fires to make people pay attention and listen to me"), peer favour (e.g., "I thought my friends would like me more if I started fires"), presence of auditory hallucinations (e.g., "I started fires because a voice outside my head told me to"), depression (e.g., "I felt so miserable I had to start fires"), anger (e.g., "I started fires because I was cross with people"), and demand escape or avoidance (e.g., "I started fires to get out of going somewhere or doing something"). All items are rated as either "usually," "sometimes," or "never" true.

Murphy and Clare (1996) tested the reliability of the FAS using a sample of ten adults (7 men, 3 women) with mild intellectual disabilities who were inpatients at a regional learning disability service. The FAS was completed on two separate occasions by nine of the ten participants to establish test-retest reliability. Murphy and Clare found better test-retest reliability for pre-firesetting factors ($k = .65$) than post-firesetting factors ($k = .39$)

suggesting that the FAS may be most useful for assessing factors preceding incidents of firesetting.

Fire Setting Scale (Gannon & Barrowcliffe, 2012)

The FSS is a 20-item self-report measure developed to assess community adults' self-reported interest in fire and engagement in antisocial behaviour—two key factors found to be associated with deliberate firesetting in apprehended populations (Gannon & Pina, 2010). Items within the FSS were derived from the empirical literature on adult and adolescent firesetting and are sub-divided into two 10-item subscales: one assessing fire interest (e.g., "I find fire intriguing" and "I get excited thinking about fire") and the other antisocial behaviour (e.g., "I like to engage in acts that are dangerous" and "I am a rule breaker"). Responders rate how much each statement is like them on a 7-point scale (1 = not at all like me, 7 = very strongly like me), and a score for each of the subscales is computed.

The FSS has been validated with UK samples of un-apprehended firesetting individuals (i.e., those in the community whose self-reported firesetting has not been detected) and non-firesetting participants, with good internal validity ($\alpha = .86$) and test-retest reliability ($r = .86$) reported (Gannon & Barrowcliffe, 2012). It has also been shown to be able to discriminate between firesetting individuals and non-firesetting individuals, with those who hold a self-reported history of firesetting scoring significantly higher on the measure than non-firesetting individuals (Barrowcliffe & Gannon, 2015, 2016; Barrowcliffe et al., in press; Gannon & Barrowcliffe, 2012). However, the measure has yet to be validated with apprehended firesetting populations or with other cultural groups, and clinical cut-off scores (i.e., the boundary point at which scores are considered to be in the "clinical" or "problematic" range) have yet to be developed.

Fire Proclivity Scale (Gannon & Barrowcliffe, 2012)

The FPS was developed alongside the FSS to assess individuals' interest, arousal to fire, and general antisocial behaviour, as well as behavioural intentions to engage in firesetting. Modelled on Bohner et al.'s (1998) Rape Proclivity Scale, the FPS consists of six hypothetical scenarios depicting a series of incidents of intentional firesetting. Respondents read each scenario and then indicate on a series of 5-point scales (1) their fascination with the fire in the scenario (e.g., "In this situation, how fascinated would you be by the fire?"; 1 = not at all fascinated, 5 = very strongly fascinated), (2) their behavioural propensity to engage in the same way described (e.g., "In this situation could you see yourself doing the same?"; 1 = would definitely not have done the same, 5 = would definitely have done the same), (3) their arousal to the fire in the scenario (e.g., "In this situation, how much would you have enjoyed watching the fire"; 1 = would not enjoy it at all, 5 = would greatly enjoy it), and (4) their enjoyment of antisocial behaviour (e.g., "Imagine that someone [e.g., a passer-by] had seen you light the fire. In this situation, how much would you have enjoyed watching their reaction?"; 1 = would not enjoy it at all, 5 = would greatly enjoy it). A score is generated for each of the four subscales as well as a total score of firesetting proclivity.

Similar to the FSS, the FPS was developed and validated with a UK community sample of un-apprehended firesetting and non-firesetting adults. The authors of the measure report that the FPS has good psychometric properties (i.e., internal consistency [α = .82], test re-test reliability [r = .88]) and that the total score and three of the subscales (e.g., fire interest, arousal to fire, and behavioural propensity) showed good discriminant validity between those who had set fires and those who had not (Gannon & Barrowcliffe, 2012). Further, scores on the behavioural propensity subscale were found to significantly predict firesetting or non-firesetting status (Gannon & Barrowcliffe, 2012). Thus, the FPS appears to represent a reasonably reliable and valid measure of factors associated with un-apprehended firesetting. However, similarly to the FSS, this measure has not been validated with apprehended firesetting adults or outside of the UK context.

Four Factor Fire Scale (Ó Ciardha et al., 2015b, 2015c)

The FFFS combines items from three pre-existing measures, the Fire Interest Rating Scale (Murphy & Clare, 1996), the Fire Attitude Scale (Muckley, 1997), and the Identification with Fire Questionnaire (Gannon et al., 2011). The Fire Interest Rating Scale (Murphy & Clare, 1996) consists of 14 fire-related scenarios (e.g., "watching a house burn down"), which respondents rate on a 7-point scale ("1 = upsetting/frightening," "7 = exciting, fun, or lovely"). The Fire Attitude Scale (Muckley, 1997) is a measure of fire supportive attitudes (e.g., "setting just a small fire can make you feel a lot better"). It consists of 20 items rated on a 5-point scale (1 = strongly disagree, 5 = strongly agree). The Identification with Fire Questionnaire (Gannon et al., 2011) consists of 10 items rated on a 5-point scale (1 = strongly disagree, 5 = strongly agree) that measure identification and affinity with fire (e.g., "fire is an important part of my identity").

To ascertain whether these measures appraise three distinct constructs, Ó Ciardha et al. (2015b) conducted a factor analysis of items across the three measures using data from a sample of 234 adult male prisoners (117 firesetting, 117 non-firesetting). A five-factor solution was initially identified; however, this was later revised to four factors, as one factor (everyday fire interest) was found not to discriminate between firesetting and non-firesetting individuals (Ó Ciardha et al., 2015c). The final four factors (or subscales) represent the themes of *identification with fire, serious fire interest, fire safety awareness*, and *normalisation of firesetting*. Clinical cut-off scores have been developed for the FFFS for prison populations (women and men, male youths) and forensic mental health samples (women and men), providing clinicians with an indication as to whether a client's responding is closer to the mean of a firesetting or non-firesetting population and therefore a key area for treatment. However, the samples with which the FFFS was validated are small and highly selective, and clinical cut-off scores for individuals with intellectual and developmental difficulties are lacking. Further, none of the measures underpinning the FFFS have been validated outside of the UK.

Firesetting Questionnaire (Gannon et al., in preparation)

The FQ represents a recent development in assessing attitudes, interests, and associations with fire. The FQ was developed from a factor analysis of 171 questions, including items from the original five-factor solution of the FFFS (Ó Ciardha et al., 2015b), the fire interest subscale of the FSS (Gannon & Barrowcliffe, 2012), and 117 new questions informed by

Butler and Gannon's (2015) conceptualisation of firesetting scripts as well as the M-TTAF (Gannon et al., 2012). Factor analysis using data from 1,402 community participants (137 firesetters, 1,265 non-firesetters) generated a 91-item scale organised into eight factors termed *firesetting as normal, identification with fire, fire interest, fire safety, pathological fire interest, coping using fire, fire is a powerful messenger*, and *fascination with fire paraphernalia*. All factors had acceptable to excellent internal consistency ($\alpha = .71–.95$) and discriminated between individuals who reported having set fires and those who did not. Following initial scale development, the FQ was validated with a further sample of imprisoned men who had set deliberate fires ($n = 49$), imprisoned men who had engaged in other types of offences ($n = 62$), and a non-forensic community control group ($n = 30$). FQ factors were found to measure a common (albeit multi-dimensional) psychological construct of firesetting propensity, with individuals who had set fires scoring higher than prison *and* community controls on *identification with fire* (e.g., I need fire in my life), *coping using fire* (e.g., I set fires to unwind), and *fire is a powerful messenger* (e.g., Fire will get a person what they want) whilst controlling for age and IQ. These differences were broad in magnitude. Whilst the FQ represents another step forward in the assessment of fire-specific factors, the measure has yet to be validated with other forensic populations (e.g., forensic mental health, intellectual and developmental disabilities) and with non-UK samples. Further, clinical cut-off scores have yet to be developed to identify levels of normative and problematic responding.

To conclude, a number of structured tools have been developed to aid the assessment of fire-specific factors in adults. Whilst these measures represent a significant development in the field, they are not without their limitations. It is therefore important that clinicians carefully consider both the aim of their assessment as well as the strengths and weaknesses of each measure when evaluating which might be best suited to supporting their assessment of an individual's firesetting. Further, given the limited reliability and validity data available for these measures and the highly selected samples that they were developed from, it is important that these are completed in conjunction with other assessments (e.g., clinical interview and review of collateral information) so as to develop a detailed understanding of these factors, as well as other fire-related factors not assessed by these measures (e.g., fire scripts and implicit theories) and if and how they are related to an individual's firesetting behaviour. A strengths-based pre-treatment assessment should also ask individuals about their individual talents, examine the individual's unique pattern of psychological strengths and vulnerabilities in relation to their offending (see Willis et al., 2013) and gather information about the individual's previous experience of groups.

Treatment of Adult Firesetting

To date, there has been a distinct lack of focus on developing, implementing, and evaluating interventions to reduce risk of firesetting in adults. A national survey of intervention providers in the UK (e.g., prisons, forensic mental health services, fire and rescue services) in 2005 found only seven services reported providing specialist interventions for adults who set deliberate fires (Palmer et al., 2005). Whilst there has been developments in treatment approaches for firesetting over the past 15 years the availability of specialist interventions for firesetting internationally remains limited (Tyler et al., 2019b). Consequently, firesetting behaviour in adults has traditionally been addressed via general interventions, either aimed at addressing offending behaviour more generally (i.e., not firesetting specific) or only one particular issue associated with the individual's firesetting (e.g., anger management, social skills, fire interest, or mental health symptoms; Gannon & Pina, 2010; Haines et al., 2006). In this section, an overview of the existing evidence for both generalist and specialist interventions for adult deliberate firesetting is provided and effectiveness data for each considered.

Generalist Interventions

There have been a handful of published reports on the effectiveness of general interventions with adults who have set fires. These predominantly consist of single-case studies (e.g., Ashworth et al., 2017; Delshadian, 2003; Lande, 1980; Parks et al., 2005; Royer et al., 1971) or small sample group evaluations (e.g., Rice & Chaplin, 1979). Two of the earliest case studies describe the use of conditioning techniques to reduce interest and arousal to fire. Royer et al. (1971) describe the effects of aversive conditioning therapy for a man with a diagnosis of schizophrenia and a history of repeat firesetting. Treatment consisted of two phases: in phase one, the patient was presented with a series of cards to read which contained either neutral words or fire words (i.e., "fire" and "flame"). Electric shocks were administered to the hands of the patient each time he read the fire words. As no behavioural change was observed following phase one, phase two of treatment was implemented in which the patient was instructed to set light to pieces of tissue and then throw them into a pan of water. This process was repeated 20 times. For the first three sessions, electric shocks were administered each time the flame of the match touched the tissue. Following the third session, shocks were administered when the patient ignited the match. Increased latencies were observed before lighting the match following the third session of treatment; however, further firesetting occurred (after approximately nine sessions of treatment), and additional booster sessions were provided following each incident. The authors report that following the sixth booster session no further firesetting was observed over a 4-year follow-up.

In the second study, Lande (1980) describes the use of orgasmic reconditioning and covert sensitisation with a 20-year-old man who had set fires in the context of sexual arousal. Treatment consisted of two phases: four sessions of orgasmic reconditioning followed by three sessions of covert sensitisation. During the orgasmic reconditioning sessions, the participant was asked to masturbate to fire images followed by images of nude females whilst imagining heterosexual activity; this cycle was repeated 15 times during each session. The patient was instructed to withhold orgasm until the 15th pairing when he was allowed four minutes to ejaculate to the nude female image. During the covert sensitisation sessions, the participant was asked to masturbate to fire images whilst listening to a "highly unpleasant scene" being described based on the consequences of their firesetting; this cycle was repeated three times each session. Sexual interest was assessed using heart rate monitoring, penile circumference measurement, and self-reported sexual arousal pre- and post-treatment, and then again at 4- and 9-month follow-up. Lande (1980) reports that, post-treatment, the participant showed less arousal to fire images and more arousal to nude female images on both physiological and self-report measures, which was maintained at 4- and 9-month follow-up. No further incidents of firesetting were reported at 9-month follow-up.

Rice and Chaplin (1979) examined the effectiveness of group-based social skills training compared with non-directive group psychotherapy, with a sample of ten male maximum-security hospital patients. All participants had a conviction for an arson-related offence, and five had a mild or borderline intellectual disability. The study utilised a cross-over design whereby participants completed both interventions, with one group completing the social skills training first and the other the non-directive group psychotherapy. Outcomes for both interventions were assessed via facilitator-rated role plays and multiple-choice assertiveness questionnaires, which were completed before the first treatment, between treatments, and following completing both treatments. Rice and Chaplin (1979) report that participants' ratings on the role plays significantly improved following completion of social skills training compared with non-directive group psychotherapy. Further, following treatment, eight participants were discharged from hospital, and no known or suspected fires were reported at 12-month follow-up.

Delshadian (2003) describes a case study of the use of art therapy with a woman with a history of repeat firesetting and self-injury in a UK prison. The focus of the art therapy sessions was to explore the participant's firesetting and self-harm and the reasons underpinning them using art to mediate between verbal and non-verbal ways of thinking and behaving. In addition to attending sessions with an art therapist, the participant was also provided with art materials and a diary to use between sessions. Delshadian reports that the participant's firesetting and self-harm reduced during therapy. However, longer term treatment outcomes are not reported.

Parks et al. (2005) describe a case study of pharmacological treatment for a 20-year-old man admitted to a UK psychiatric hospital, who met the diagnostic criteria for pyromania. Treatment consisted of 300 mg (increased to 800 mg) of anticonvulsant sodium valproate and 10 mg of olanzapine. Neuropsychological tests assessing attention, verbal and visual memory, executive functioning, and visuospatial and language skills were administered at admission and again 5 months later. The frequency of aggressive incidents was also recorded. Parks et al. (2005) report that at 5-month follow-up, the participant showed an improvement across all cognitive assessments, but her visuospatial and language skills remained the same. They also reported a significant negative correlation between the number of aggressive incidents and length of admission. Three years post-discharge, no further firesetting incidents had been reported.

More recently, Ashworth et al. (2017) presented a case study on the effectiveness of an adapted dialectical behavioural therapy (DBT) programme (*I Can Feel Good*; Ingamells & Morrissey, 2014) for a man with a mild intellectual disability and a history of deliberate firesetting. *I Can Feel Good* consists of group sessions that cover mindfulness, emotional regulation, distress tolerance, and interpersonal effectiveness, alongside individual therapy sessions focused on cognitive and behavioural change strategies. Ashworth et al. (2017) report that the client in the case study attended 38 of the 47 groups sessions, with the final nine sessions being completed individually. Within-treatment change was assessed using pre- and post-treatment psychometric assessments that tapped into the four key areas of treatment. Ashworth et al. (2017) report mixed treatment outcomes, with the participant reporting improved application of mindfulness techniques; however, little change was observed on self-reported emotion regulation strategies, coping strategies, and interpersonal reactions. No firesetting specific outcomes were collected, so it is unclear whether the intervention was effective in reducing reoffending.

Specialist Interventions

In addition to generalist interventions, there have also been several reports of more specialist interventions for firesetting. Again, these predominantly consist of single-case descriptions or small sample group studies. Published reports of specialist interventions can be broadly grouped as either adopting a cognitive analytic approach to therapy or a cognitive behavioural orientation.

Cognitive analytic–oriented interventions. Several detailed clinical case descriptions have been published on the use of cognitive analytic therapy (CAT) protocols with adults who have set fires with a diagnosis of a learning disability or borderline personality disorder (e.g., Clayton, 2000; Pollock, 2006). However, few evaluation data have been published on the effectiveness of this approach in reducing firesetting adults' treatment needs and reoffending. One of the few published evaluations of a CAT-informed therapy for firesetting was reported by Annesley et al. (2017). Annesley et al. describe the implementation and evaluation of two firesetting interventions for adult women in a UK high-secure hospital: the Arson Treatment Group Programme (ATGP) and the Arson Treatment Individual Programme (ATIP). Both interventions combined CAT and cognitive behavioural approaches and covered modules on *dangerousness of firesetting, coping and social skills, trauma, self-esteem and self-awareness*, and *relapse prevention*. The ATGP comprised weekly group sessions and weekly or fortnightly individual sessions for 18 months. The ATIP was designed for patients who were unable to attend group treatment due to risk issues and consisted of 32 individual sessions. Twenty-two women commenced treatment, 14 in the ATGP and 9 in the ATIP. Nine women completed the ATGP, and six completed the ATIP. Participants attending both interventions completed a battery of psychometrics pre- and post-treatment. The psychometric battery is reported to have changed between each round of delivery; however, they broadly assessed motivations for firesetting, problem solving, coping, emotional regulation, self-esteem, and impression management. Annesley et al. (2017) report that participants who attended both interventions demonstrated improvements in their pre- and post-treatment scores across the majority of measures based on mean score differences. However, no statistical comparisons were undertaken due to the small sample size; thus, it is unclear if the changes observed were statistically or clinically meaningful. Further, the lack of reoffending data and a comparison group means it is not possible to draw any conclusions about whether CAT-informed firesetting interventions are effective in reducing firesetting reoffending or if they are as effective or more effective than other therapeutic approaches (e.g., cognitive behavioural therapy [CBT]).

Cognitive behavioural interventions. Meta-analyses have consistently indicated that CBT interventions have a positive effect on recidivism for a range of offending behaviours, with an average reduction in reoffending reported of approximately 25% (Lipsey et al., 2007). Despite the evidence for offence-specific CBT interventions, there are only a small number of published accounts on the use of offence-specific CBT for deliberate firesetting.

In one of the earliest published evaluations, Clare et al. (1992) present a case study of a 23-year-old male patient with a mild intellectual disability and a history of making hoax calls to the fire and rescue service and deliberate firesetting. A tailored package of treatment was developed that followed a cognitive behavioural framework. The treatment plan was provided over an 18-month period and included progressive muscle relaxation, social skills training, coping strategies training, assertiveness training, surgery for facial disfigurement, "assisted" covert sensitisation for fire interest, and graded exposure to fire-related paraphernalia. Clare et al. (1992) report that no hoax calls were made, and no fires were set during the patient's admission. Further, they report that there was no evidence of further firesetting or hoax calls at 30-month follow-up. Although the reported treatment gains are encouraging, it is important to note the treatment plan described by Clare et al. was very much tailored to the specific needs of the client and involved a suite of interventions delivered at different stages. Further, the absence of outcome measures limits the conclusions that can be drawn about the impact of the treatment plan on psychological factors associated with firesetting or which component of treatment contributed to behavioural change.

Hall (1995) describes a specialist group-based intervention that was developed for men and women with a history of repetitive firesetting at a UK high-secure psychiatric hospital. The intervention is reported to consist of weekly group sessions and ran for a minimum of 1 year. The intervention was underpinned by cognitive behavioural principles and Jackson et al.'s (1987) functional analysis theory (see Chapter 3). Treatment targeted *coping, self-awareness and self-esteem, family and relationships*, and *beliefs and knowledge about fire*. A battery of psychometric measures was administered pre- and post-treatment that assessed fear of negative evaluation, suggestibility, social acceptance and distress, assertiveness, and social desirability. However, due to small numbers ($n = 7$), no evaluation data were reported.

Swaffer et al. (2001) describe a similarly structured group-based intervention for firesetting to that of Hall (1995). However, Swaffer et al.'s offence-specific treatment package was developed and delivered in another UK high-secure psychiatric hospital. The intervention was offered as a mixed-sex programme to 10 patients (4 men, 6 women), the majority of whom had an index offence of arson. The intervention consisted of both weekly group sessions and monthly individual sessions and ran over a period of 16 months. Similar to Hall (1995), Swaffer et al.'s intervention was underpinned by Jackson et al.'s (1987) functional analysis theory, with modules focusing on *dangers of fire, coping skills, insight and self-awareness*, and *relapse prevention*. A standardised battery of psychometrics was administered pre- and post-treatment that assessed participants' motivations for firesetting, fire interest, assertiveness, self-esteem, fear of negative evaluation, problem solving, anger, depression, and readiness to change. Further, facilitators rated participants at the end of each session on their attentiveness, communication, alertness, co-cooperativeness, appropriateness and level of disclosure during the group. At the time of reporting, participants had only completed two of the four modules within the intervention. Treatment effectiveness was therefore presented via a descriptive mid-treatment case study, highlighting the positive progress of one patient. However, no post-treatment data are reported, so it is not possible to draw any conclusions as to whether the observed progress translated to measurable psychological or behavioural change following treatment completion.

As part of their national survey, Palmer et al. (2005) provide a descriptive case example of an unpublished cognitive behavioural intervention designed and delivered by clinical staff at Broadmoor, a UK high-secure hospital. The intervention included 21 to 27 weekly group sessions, dependent on group size, and aimed to increase participants' understanding of their firesetting, the dangers of fire, and how to manage firesetting risk in the future. Single-sex groups were offered for both male and female patients with a history of repeat firesetting as an adult. At the time of publishing, Palmer et al. (2005) reported that 70 patients had been referred to the intervention, and 11 had completed the programme (one male group, one female group). Pre- versus post-treatment change was assessed using a battery of psychometrics that examined fire interest, motivations for firesetting, blame attribution, locus of control, anger, self-esteem, social avoidance and distress, and fear of negative evaluation. However, no evaluation of the intervention had taken place due to the low number of completed pre- and post-treatment psychometrics.

Hall et al. (2005) provide a practice-based account of a group firesetting intervention for patients with an intellectual disability, developed and delivered at a UK medium-secure hospital. The intervention was cognitive behavioural in orientation and consisted of 16 weekly sessions that aimed to help participants identify risk factors associated with their firesetting and to develop alternative coping strategies to reduce their risk of reoffending. Outcome measures were completed pre- and post-treatment that assessed blame attribution, self-assessed risk, fire interest, motivations for firesetting, and self-esteem. Whilst Hall et al. (2005) describe in some detail the characteristics of six male participants and their pre-treatment assessment scores, no quantitative analysis of within-treatment change on the pre-and post-treatment psychometrics are reported.

One specialist intervention that has received quantitative evaluation is the Northgate Firesetters Treatment Programme (NFTP; Taylor et al., 2002). The NFTP is a 40- to 45-session group intervention for men and women with intellectual disabilities. Similar to other specialist interventions, the NFTP adopts a functional analytic approach to treatment (i.e., Jackson et al., 1987) and consists of sessions on *life mapping* (e.g., exploring life events, systems, and schemas), *offence analysis, self-esteem, fire safety education, communication, coping and emotion management*, and *relapse prevention* (Taylor & Thorne, 2013). A series of clinical outcome measures was completed by group members pre- and post-treatment that measured their interests and attitudes towards fire, goal attainment, anger, depression, and self-esteem. Taylor and colleagues (2002, 2004, 2006) examined the effectiveness of the NFTP by comparing pre- and post-treatment scores on each of the clinical outcome measures for two groups of male patients ($n = 8$) and one group of female patients ($n = 6$). Taylor and colleagues (2002, 2004, 2006) reported significant pre- versus post-treatment improvements across all outcome measures except for the depression measure. Further, Taylor (2014) reported on a post-hoc service evaluation that examined the progression and reoffending rates of 24 men and women (16 men, 8 women) who had completed the NFTP, drawn from file data, over an average follow-up period of 8 years and 10 months (range = 4 years to 12 years, 9 months). Of the 24 treatment completers, 17 were now living in the community. Of those not in the community, one was reported to be in prison, four remained in hospital, and two were deceased. In terms of reoffending, Taylor (2014) reports that no further arrests or convictions for firesetting were reported amongst participants. However, one participant was known to have set a fire, two were suspected of setting small fires, and two had threatened or voiced thoughts about setting fires during the follow-up period. Thus, the majority of participants were not reported to display any fire-related risk behaviours during the follow-up period. Whilst the findings from Taylor and colleagues' small-scale studies both build upon earlier descriptive case reports and provide encouraging results, the lack of a comparison group makes it difficult to determine whether this particular specialist intervention is effective.

As noted earlier, the majority of CBT interventions for deliberate firesetting have utilised Jackson et al.'s (1987) functional analytic approach to inform treatment targets. However, more recently, practitioners have adopted the more contemporary M-TTAF model (Gannon et al., 2012) to inform specialist CBT interventions for firesetting. One example of this is the Australian Centre for Arson Research and Treatment Firesetter Treatment Programme (ACART; Fritzon et al., 2013). The ACART programme is designed to address firesetting in both adolescents and adults in the community or correctional settings. It is modular in nature with individual components designed to target M-TTAF risk factors (Gannon et al., 2012) as well as fire safety education. The ACART programme adopts an individualised strengths-based approach to rehabilitation, incorporating key principles from the Risk Need Responsivity Model and the Good Lives Model (Bonta & Andrews, 2017; Ward et al., 2007) alongside a flexible delivery format so that specific areas of individual need can be effectively addressed. The ACART is subject to ongoing evaluation, and to date, 20 individuals are reported to have completed the programme, with pre- and post-treatment data collected for between 4 and 17 participants (depending on the outcome measure). Although effectiveness data for the ACART are limited, preliminary findings suggest that participants who completed both the programme and the pre- and post-treatment psychometrics have made small but positive improvements across the majority of treatment domains (Fritzon et al., 2022).

In addition to the ACART programme, two specialist CBT interventions have been developed in the UK: The Firesetting Intervention Programme for Prisoners (FIPP; Gannon, 2012, 2017) and the Firesetting Intervention Programme for Mentally Disordered Offenders (FIP-MO; Gannon & Lockerbie, 2011, 2012, 2014, 2017). The FIPP and FIP-MO are sister programmes designed specifically for adults who have a history of deliberate firesetting or fire-related risk behaviours. The programmes are underpinned by contemporary theories of rehabilitation (e.g., Good Lives Model, Ward et al., 2006; Risk Need Responsivity Model; Bonta & Andrews, 2017) with treatment targets derived from the critical risk factors outlined within the M-TTAF (Gannon et al., 2012): *fire-related factors* (e.g., interests and associations with fire, fire scripts, fire safety awareness), *offence-supportive cognition* (e.g., attitudes that support firesetting or general offending), *emotional/self-regulation* (e.g., coping, mood and anger management), and *social competence* (e.g., problem solving, communication, self-esteem). The programmes incorporate CBT principles alongside strong psychotherapeutic elements to support self-reflection, healthy social and emotional expression, and a strong therapeutic alliance. Areas of treatment need are addressed within the programme through a range of activities including interactive exercises, group discussions and presentations, experiential tasks, psychoeducation sessions, role play, conditioning techniques, and out-of-group skills practice. Participants are encouraged throughout the programmes to apply the skills and coping strategies learnt to factors associated with their own firesetting and are supported to develop a detailed safety plan for the future.

Both the FIPP and FIP-MO have been evaluated as part of multi-site research projects to establish the effectiveness of the programmes in reducing psychological factors associated with firesetting. Both evaluations adopted a quasi-experimental design and compared pre- and post-treatment psychometric scores of programme completers to that of a comparison group, who were considered treatment eligible but had not completed the FIPP or FIP-MO. Pre- and post-treatment psychometric measures assessed each of the key treatment targets within the programme (e.g., fire-related factors, offence-supportive attitudes, social competency, and self/emotional regulation) as well as social desirability. The FIPP evaluation was conducted by Gannon et al. (2015) over a 24-month period. FIPP groups ran across two UK adult male prisons ($n = 54$), and comparison participants ($n = 45$) were recruited from five other UK adult male establishments. The FIP-MO evaluation was conducted by Tyler et al. (2018). Fifty-two men and women who had completed the FIP-MO and 40 comparison participants were recruited from across 26 secure mental health hospitals in the UK. Both the FIPP and FIP-MO evaluations found that, relative to the comparison groups, participants who completed the programmes made significant improvements on fire-related factors (e.g., attitudes, interests and associations with fire) and anger regulation or expression. Further, effect size calculations indicated that FIPP and FIP-MO participants made larger improvements pre- versus post-treatment compared with the comparison group across the majority of outcome measures. As part of the FIPP evaluation, Gannon et al. followed participants for 3 months post-treatment and repeated the psychometric measures to see if treatment effects were maintained. Gannon et al. report that all improvements observed in FIPP participants immediately post-treatment were still present at 3-month follow-up. These findings suggest that the FIPP and FIP-MO are effective in reducing the psychological risk factors associated with deliberate firesetting. However, due to the absence of recidivism data, it is not possible to conclude as yet whether the programmes are effective in reducing reoffending. Recidivism data is currently being collected for both FIPP and comparison participants from Gannon et al.'s study. To date, 7 years of follow-up data have been collected, with findings due to be reported in the near future.

Individualised treatment. Most published accounts of specialist interventions for deliberate firesetting have focused on group-based programmes, with only a couple reporting individualised treatment (e.g., Annesley et al., 2017; Clare et al., 1992). Group-based interventions are often offered in forensic settings as they allow for offence-specific treatment to be provided to multiple clients simultaneously, providing both a fiscally and therapeutically effective way of delivering treatment (Duggan, 2008; Rees-Jones, 2011). However, it is important to acknowledge that group-based therapy may not always be feasible or appropriate for a variety of reasons. For example, individual client factors (e.g., complex mental health needs, difficulties with functioning in a group setting, and risk issues), clinical need (e.g., not enough people for a group), organisational factors, and ethical issues (e.g., delaying treatment) may all determine whether individualised treatment is more appropriate (Davies, 2019). There is a distinct lack of research examining the role of treatment modality on therapeutic outcomes in forensic settings, however, findings from the wider psychotherapy literature suggest both modalities can be equally effective in bringing about change (Davies, 2019).

Annesley et al. (2017) is the only published account of specialist treatment for firesetting that reports outcomes for both group and individualised delivery. Although they did not make direct comparisons between group and individual participants, Annesley et al. report similar treatment outcomes for both modalities even though the group programme was much higher in dosage than the individualised programme (18 months of weekly group sessions versus 8 months of individual sessions). The FIPP programme is also currently being evaluated as part of a multi-site research project comparing the effects of group and individual delivery (Sambrooks & Tyler, 2019). Whilst it is not possible at this stage to determine the average dosage of individual FIPP treatment, anecdotally, practitioners using the programme on a one-to-one basis have reported delivering weekly 1-hour sessions that focus on the group content and adapt group exercises to more individually focused discussions. Therefore, although empirical evidence of individualised treatment for firesetting is currently lacking, the initial findings reported above suggest that some existing group interventions may lend themselves to be adapted to individual delivery.

Conclusions, Ways of Working, and Future Directions

Whilst there has been much progress over the last 15 years, evidence-based protocols for assessment and treatment of deliberate firesetting are still in their infancy. The assessment tools currently available to measure fire-related factors (e.g., interests, attitudes, motivations, and associations with fire) provide practitioners with a series of structured instruments to support their assessment of key factors that research suggests are associated with deliberate firesetting. That said, due to the limited reliability and validity data available, it is important for practitioners to carefully consider the focus, strengths, and weaknesses of each measure when evaluating which one might best aid their assessment of an individual's firesetting. At present, the FFFS (Ó Ciardha et al., 2015c) and FQ (Gannon et al., in preparation) represent the most rigorously tested measures of fire-related factors with apprehended populations. However, it is important to recognise that whilst relatively good psychometric properties are reported, it is unclear whether these, as well as the other tools discussed, are (1) appropriate outside of the settings which they were developed and (2) appropriate for use within different cultural contexts (e.g., whether individual items reflect attitudes, interests, and associations with fire across cultures). It is therefore suggested that when formulating firesetting behaviour, practitioners supplement any measures used with clinical interview data and collateral information. Future research would benefit from exploring the properties of existing assessment tools across different cultural contexts to further establish their validity as well as their cultural sensitivity and appropriateness.

As highlighted earlier in this chapter, there have been very few published evaluations on the effectiveness of specialist interventions for adult firesetting. Whilst there is an emerging body of research with some positive findings, there is still a need for more high-quality evaluation studies. Existing research suggests that offence-specific CBT is an effective therapeutic approach for reducing psychological factors associated with deliberate firesetting. However, it is important to note that the majority of published accounts report on treatment provided for (1) individuals with a history of repeat firesetting, (2) group-based interventions and, (3) CBT-oriented interventions. Thus, it is difficult to draw conclusions about the effectiveness of specialist interventions for adults who have set a single fire, interventions delivered on an individual basis, and specialist interventions using alternative therapeutic approaches (e.g., fire safety education, CAT, DBT).

Longitudinal evaluations of the FIPP and FIP-MO are currently underway examining the effectiveness of the programmes in reducing reconviction, the effect of modality (e.g., group versus individual) on treatment outcomes, and any effects of treatment non-completion; however, the results of these studies are not due for several years (Sambrooks & Tyler, 2019). Future evaluations of specialist firesetting interventions would benefit from examining any differences in treatment outcomes for different characteristics (e.g., one-time versus repeat firesetting, age and gender) as well as the impact of interventions on reoffending, to further our understanding of effective rehabilitation approaches with this population and "what works best for whom." Due to reporting issues associated with firesetting offences, future evaluations would also benefit from incorporating a range of long-term outcome measures, for example, reconviction data, unofficial reoffending data, self-reported offending, and progress following treatment completion (e.g., move to lower security, discharge, housing, and employment; Friendship et al., 2003). Using an integrated model of evaluation would provide a range of possible outcomes through which to assess intervention effectiveness and potentially provide a more accurate picture of treatment efficacy (Friendship et al., 2003). Finally, whilst offence-specific CBT currently shows the most promise for addressing firesetting in adults, it is important to note that there are few evaluations of interventions utilising different therapeutic approaches. To further our understanding on "what works best for whom," evaluations of other promising treatment approaches should be considered. Future research in these areas will enable the continued development of an evidence base for effective assessment and treatment with adults who have set deliberate fires.

7

Engaging and Working Therapeutically with Individuals Who Have Set Deliberate Fires: A Strengths-Based Approach

Over the past two decades, treatment delivery for offending behaviour in general has become increasingly strengths-based (de Ruiter, 2018; Tyler et al., 2020; Willis et al., 2013). Collaborative and strengths-based interventions for offending behaviour typically involve identifying and working with an individual's competencies and strengths to promote desistance. Strengths-based psychological approaches offer a positive alternative to problem-based or risk-focused approaches, which tend to pathologize individuals, focusing predominantly on risk and its avoidance (see Fogarty et al., 2018; Ward & Stewart, 2003). Examples of strengths-based treatment approaches for offending include avoiding disempowering and pathologizing labels such as "offender" (Willis, 2018; Willis & Letourneau, 2018), adopting positively directed approach goals to encourage genuine engagement in treatment and motivation to live an offence-free life (Mann et al., 2004), and examining how a person can further improve their competencies and talents to improve life quality whilst in turn strengthening desistance (Ward & Stewart, 2003; Willis et al., 2013).

A widely used strengths-based rehabilitation framework for treating individuals who have offended is that of the Good Lives Model (Ward, 2010; Ward et al., 2007; Ward & Stewart, 2003). In brief, this framework states that offending behaviour occurs when individuals do not have the skills and opportunities to live a rewarding or "good" life characterised by key experiences or "primary human goods" such as *relatedness* (i.e., the need to hold affectionate bonds with others through friendships, romance, and platonic relationships), *autonomy* (i.e., the need to direct one's own life through the development and achievement of goals), and *inner peace* (i.e., the need to remain free from stress and inner turmoil; see Ward, 2010 for definitions and examples of all ten experiences). The Good Lives Model's popularity seems to rest on its theoretical assumption that criminogenic and human needs are inextricably related (Ward, 2010). Proponents of the Good Lives Model view the therapeutic promotion of an individual's skills and opportunities to lead a good life as, in turn, reducing their risk and attendant potential to offend (see Ward, 2010; Ward et al., 2007). In contrast, risk-focused rehabilitation (i.e., the Risk-Need-Responsivity model; Andrews & Bonta, 2010; Bonta & Andrews, 2017) appears to view individuals who have offended via a deficit or problem-based lens and focuses on reducing an individual's risk with little emphasis on their overall life quality (Ward, 2010).

In this chapter, we assume that readers are reasonably familiar with the Good Lives Model of rehabilitation as we walk readers through our strengths-based approaches to engaging and working therapeutically with individuals who have set fires. For those who feel that they would like a better grounding in strengths-based psychological approaches and the Good Lives Model prior to reading this chapter, we refer them to Ward (2010), Ward and Stewart (2003), Willis et al. (2013), and Willis et al. (2016).

In the sections that follow, we present common challenges that we have faced in recruiting and facilitating group based treatment for individuals who have set fires in relation to the Firesetting Intervention Programme for Prisoners (FIPP; Gannon, 2012, 2017) and the Firesetting Intervention Programme for Mentally Disordered Offenders (FIP-MO; Gannon & Lockerbie, 2011, 2012, 2014, 2017). While we acknowledge that a lot of treatment for individuals who have set fires is conducted individually, the developing evidence base on effectiveness of treatment for individuals who have set fires is, at present, group based (see Gannon et al., 2015; Tyler et al., 2018). Thus, until further evidence becomes available, group-based treatment should be the model of choice for treating individuals who have set fires where possible. However, readers will find that many of the themes raised in this chapter are equally applicable to individualised treatment.

Who Should Receive Treatment for Firesetting?

Our description of the revised Multi-Trajectory Theory of Adult Firesetting (M-TTAF) in Chapter 3—particularly Tier 2—highlights the variety of individuals expected to receive treatment for firesetting. Perhaps the least surprising of these are individuals who hold some level of inappropriate interest in fire (i.e., the fire interest or multi-faceted trajectories). Both fire interest and multi-faceted individuals require treatment aimed at reducing their inappropriate interest in fire. For multi-faceted individuals, however, this treatment needs to be combined with work examining and reshaping their antisocial attitudes and values.

As a treatment provider, it is relatively common to come across individuals who have set fires in an attempt to self-harm, suicide, or elicit help from others (i.e., M-TTAF Tier 2 emotionally expressive trajectory), particularly in mental health settings with patients characterised by borderline personality disorder. Such individuals are likely to require support with their communication skills and distress tolerance but also require fire-specific work to tackle their preference to misuse fire as a tool for self-harm (i.e., a *fire coping script*; see Chapter 3) or to cry for help (i.e., *fire is a powerful messenger of distress* script; see Chapter 3). It has been less common, in our practice, to come across individuals who have set fires in an attempt to gain recognition and approval from others (e.g., M-TTAF Tier 2 need for recognition trajectory). These individuals are likely to display very good self-regulation skills yet have not been able to meet their need for approval in conventional ways. Such individuals are likely to require support to gain such approval pro-socially.

A very common subtype of firesetter concerns those who set fires to gain revenge or retribution and have problems with their anger regulation (i.e., the M-TTAF Tier 2 grievance trajectory; see also Barnoux & Gannon, 2013). Such individuals may target the property (e.g., residence or business) of a person or persons perceived to have wronged them either with or without their target inside and are likely to require significant input regarding self/emotional regulation as well as work aimed at restructuring any fire-aggression fusion script that has led to fire being chosen as the tool for gaining revenge.

Individuals described by the M-TTAF's Tier 2 antisocial trajectory have historically been difficult to justify providing fire-specific treatment for. This is because their key critical risk factor clusters around antisocial cognition and values. As a result, their offending history tends to be both extensive and varied, with firesetting featuring only sporadically or very little. In the original M-TTAF, Gannon et al. (2012) proposed that fire came to be misused by individuals following this trajectory simply because they were impulsive, and fire happened to be at hand. In other words, antisocial trajectory individuals were hypothesised to grab their lighter or other fire-starting materials in the moment to meet various needs such as covering up a crime just committed, alleviating boredom, or creating excitement. In the early days of providing the FIPP (Gannon, 2012; Gannon & Lockerbie, 2017), we wondered whether such antisocial individuals really needed FIPP. After assessing a number of these individuals, however, it soon became apparent that antisocial trajectory individuals tend to misuse fire because they have developed a set of inappropriate cognitive scripts around when and how fire should be used in the context of antisocial behaviour (see Butler & Gannon, 2015). Such individuals are likely to hold entrenched cognitions that favour fire use to cover up another crime (i.e., *fire is the best way to destroy evidence script*; Butler & Gannon, 2015) or send a powerful message of revenge indirectly (i.e., *fire-aggression fusion script*; Gannon et al., 2012), so treating and reconstructing these scripts is critical. Our amended M-TTAF Tier 2 (see Chapter 3) highlights the potential existence of such scripts for antisocial individuals who have set fires. Consequently, setting up a treatment group for firesetting—particularly in the prison context—is likely to include men (and sometimes women) who are primarily antisocial and do not view themselves as requiring treatment for firesetting.

Group Composition

When assessing participants for group work in firesetting, we have found it beneficial to have as diverse a group as possible in relation to the M-TTAF trajectories outlined earlier and in Chapter 3. While empirical research is a long way off being able to pinpoint which group compositions are most likely to be beneficial for treatment outcome (see Harkins & Beech, 2007 for a review relating to sexual offence treatment), our clinical experience suggests diversity to be beneficial (see also Cowburn, 1990). We believe that diverse group membership provides key opportunities for group members to learn from varied viewpoints. It also provides each group member with numerous opportunities for support from group members who are likely to vary extensively on interpersonal style and skills. When considering group composition, if selections can be made, we advise ensuring that the group is not too heavily weighted towards a particular trajectory since this may dilute the experience of appropriate peer challenge (e.g., too many antisocial trajectory individuals may support one another's antisocial attitudes and values). Related to this, we recommend that only one or two individuals who deny having committed their firesetting offence(s) (see later) are included within each group. This balances group composition, ensuring that individuals do not reinforce each other's denial and preoccupation with the criminal justice system throughout treatment.

A group diverse in gender, however, is not recommended. This is because women who have set fires—similarly to other women who have offended—tend to have significant victimisation histories that are likely to have featured men as perpetrators (Gannon, 2010; Hall, 1995; Tyler et al., 2014). Consequently, requiring women to attend a group in which they are expected to reflect openly with men regarding past themes relevant to their firesetting could potentially be retraumatising (see Trauma).

Common Fears and Apprehensions Regarding Firesetting Treatment

Firesetting-Specific Themes

Numerous firesetting-specific fears and apprehensions are displayed by individuals considering participation in treatment for firesetting. The most notable, perhaps, relates to the reluctance that many potential participants appear to have about being associated with firesetting through attending a group examining this behaviour and being labelled accordingly (e.g., "I'm not going to a firesetting group; I'm not a pyro"). There does appear, at least to some degree, to be stigma attached to the criminal behaviour of firesetting. The roots of this lie in some of the earliest theoretical conceptions on the topic. These tended to link firesetting behaviour with mental health problems and compulsivity (Pritchard, 1833, as cited in Geller et al., 1997; Ray, 1844, as cited in Geller et al., 1997) as well as disturbed sexual development (Henke, 1812; Platner, 1797 as cited in Freud, 1932; Inciardi, 1970). Over the years, these links have proven difficult to shake (see Tyler & Gannon, 2012 or Ó Ciardha, 2016) with one particularly well known chart-topping song describing a "firestarter" as "infected" and "twisted" (Howlett et al., 1997). Poor mental health and some level of compulsivity are factors related to risk of firesetting (Tyler & Gannon, 2012; Walters, 2016). However, these factors are not inextricably interlinked risk factors since many firesetting individuals do not exhibit these features (see Chapter 3 or Tyler & Gannon, 2012). The link between firesetting and some sort of sexually abnormal behaviour has perhaps been most damaging in the sense that this perceived link has persisted in the absence of any strong empirical support (see Ó Ciardha, 2016, for a review).

When approaching individuals in prisons or hospitals about participating in treatment for firesetting, they sometimes present as extremely concerned regarding the sexual connotations of firesetting (e.g., "I'm not weird in a sexual way") or of being viewed as holding mental health problems (e.g., "I'm not ill"). Individuals who follow the antisocial trajectory of the M-TTAF are likely to be particularly sensitive to such connotations since they are unlikely to view themselves as holding any fire-related needs. In fact, they may argue that firesetting treatment is not required. When speaking to such individuals, it is important to reassure them that most people who enter treatment do not hold an inappropriate interest in fire and that treatment focuses on examining how fire comes to be misused. Using a strengths-based approach when speaking with potential treatment participants, we have found it helpful to use phrases such as "people who have set a fire" rather than pathologizing labels such as "firesetter" or "firestarter" that elicit negative connotations. We also tend to relabel the group name (e.g., *Offending Behaviour 3 Group*) so that use of the group name by prison or hospital staff does not elicit unnecessary stereotyping. Treatment participants can then be offered the opportunity to amend the group name according to their own particular preferences at the start of the group.

General Themes

When approaching individuals regarding their possible participation in firesetting treatment, fears often appear focused on the planned treatment being group based. For example, individuals may be reluctant to share private and potentially shaming information with individuals whom they are yet to meet (e.g., "I'm not telling a bunch of strangers about my offence and how I ended up here!") or to hear other individuals' life stories (e.g., "What would I want to hear other peoples' problems for?—I've got enough problems dealing with my own"). In our experience, these types of anxieties are typical for any form of group-based work examining offending behaviour. Understandably, individuals feel uncertainty about coming together to talk with residents from their institution about sensitive and personal information. They may even have prior negative relationships with other residents (e.g., having been bullied) and are wondering whether the group will involve this individual or individuals. It is always important to examine group members' previous relationships for any evidence of bullying prior to setting up group work. If such a relationship is detected, then steps can be made to ensure that these individuals do not attend the same group.

If the group being set up is not the first at your particular establishment, it can be very reassuring to offer potential participants with an opportunity to meet a previous group member who has successfully completed the treatment if logistically possible. This group member needs to be chosen carefully and should be someone who can talk about the group honestly, reflectively, and positively (i.e., in a strengths-based way). Another technique that we find helpful when approaching individuals to take part in either the FIPP or the FIP-MO is to reassure individuals that the group *does not* request individuals to disclose their offending behaviour. Instead, participants are invited to disclose what was happening in their lives in the *lead up* to their offending behaviour. Since the FIPP and FIP-MO are strengths-based, participants are never expected to talk about their offence or parts of their life if they do not wish to (Gannon, 2012, 2017; Gannon & Lockerbie, 2011, 2012, 2014, 2017). Typically, this particular apprehension around disclosing sensitive offence-related information stems from the fear that others in the group will make judgments about the offence and possibly even share details with others. Having a previous group member talk about these issues provides potential participants with the reassurance they need to participate in treatment. If a previous group member is not available, we find it helpful to talk to potential participants about our own experience of previous groups (i.e., group members tend to form powerful bonds and support one another; everyone tends to experience the group as being "in it together," so group members follow the rule of group confidentiality tightly). On this latter note, in all of the FIPP and FIP-MO groups that we have run since 2010, we have only experienced one group confidentiality issue. This was raised directly by a group member who was concerned that confidentiality had been breached. The individual in question who had breached confidentiality had not realised this breach until it was pointed out to him. He promptly apologised, and the group moved forward without issue.

Trauma. For some individuals, apprehension about entering a treatment group for firesetting goes beyond a basic fear of being judged. Like many individuals who enter the criminal justice system, individuals who have set fires have often experienced significant childhood and adulthood adversity characterised by abuse and significant loss (see Bell et al., 2018; Gannon & Pina, 2010). In such cases, individuals may be experiencing levels of trauma that make participation in firesetting treatment not just challenging but almost impossible and potentially retraumatising. This is particularly concerning when one considers that trauma may be an important risk factor for criminal behaviour (see Ardino, 2012 or Clark et al., 2014). Furthermore, trauma can be complex and associated with the firesetting offence itself (e.g., flashbacks of victims in the fire or of oneself being harmed in the fire). In such cases, it is important for the therapist to consider whether the planned firesetting treatment has the potential to retraumatise the individual as well as whether the individual holds a level of trauma that is likely to impede treatment engagement (i.e., being unable to process talking therapy due to trauma-related neuropsychological functioning; Beech & Fisher, 2011). In cases in which extremely high levels of trauma are apparent, it may be advisable to signpost the individual for appropriate assessment and resolution of this trauma prior to firesetting treatment (e.g., via eye movement desensitisation and reprocessing or cognitive behavioural therapy, National Institute for Health and Care Excellence, 2018; Seidler & Wagner, 2006). In cases in which lower levels of trauma are apparent, it will be possible to proceed since the FIPP and FIP-MO's strengths-based format is trauma informed. Trauma is viewed as an important experience that can help to explain relational patterns and ways of functioning that may have fostered firesetting. In this sense, the participant's previous experiences are appropriately acknowledged instead of simply focusing on the individual as an "offender" characterised by risk (see Levenson, 2014). Individuals are, however, given the choice as to what they would like to discuss in the group and are never expected to talk about aspects of their life that might potentially be retraumatising.

Denial. Sometimes individuals approached to take part in firesetting treatment are apprehensive or fearful about engaging in such a program because they deny having committed their firesetting offence(s). Such denial is relatively common amongst individuals who have offended (see Dealey, 2018). Denial appears to be socially adaptive in the sense that it provides individuals with a way of partitioning themselves from their socially harmful behaviour so that they can preserve a positive self-image, avoid uncomfortable feelings, remain supported by friends and family, and experience a sense of social belonging (Dealey, 2018; Harkins et al., 2015; Walton, 2019). Oftentimes, when approaching individuals who deny their firesetting, we find that they tend to refuse treatment because they (in our view understandably) feel that the group will have nothing to offer them. In such cases, we adopt an approach similar to that previously used by Marshall and his colleagues at Rockwood Psychological Services in their work with individuals who have sexually offended (see Marshall et al., 2001 or Ware & Marshall, 2008). That is, we inform potential participants that we would like them to join the treatment group to work on understanding how it is they came to be *accused* of a firesetting offence. We assure them that the treatment purpose will not be to challenge their denial and reassure them that many individuals who have been in a similar position to themselves have enjoyed participating in the group and experienced benefit from it. These reassurances are critical for enabling such individuals to consider participating in treatment. Allowing these individuals the time and space to consider their decision carefully is also usually well received as is offering them the option to leave the group after the first few sessions (prior to risk factors being considered) if they feel that it is not right for them.

Potential group members vary hugely on the elements of their firesetting that they recall, accept, or feel responsible for. Reassuring individuals that this is usual and that no one will be pressured regarding these issues is vital for enabling individuals to feel comfortable in taking the step towards treatment. In a small number of circumstances, individuals who deny their offence may be about to engage in an appeal process. In such circumstances, we typically wish the individual well and re-consider the individual (if appropriate) in our next round of treatment assessments following the appeal decision.

Navigating Group Work

Once an individual has agreed to partake in group treatment for firesetting or at least attend the first few sessions and an appropriate assessment has been conducted, the challenging process of group work begins. In our view, it is critical that individuals feel safe and supported within the group environment. A safe and supportive group atmosphere encourages strong group cohesiveness and expressiveness, which have been linked to both increased participation and retention in therapeutic groups more generally (Budman et al., 1993; Piper et al., 1983) as well as treatment gains in offending groups more specifically (see Beech & Hamilton-Giachritsis, 2005). Increased group cohesiveness and other helpful group processes are generally considered to be linked to a more effective therapeutic alliance (see Serran et al., 2003). Detailed information on the importance of the therapeutic alliance in offence-related treatment has been provided by Marshall and Burton (2010) and Marshall et al. (2013) and is not repeated in detail here. However, it is important to mention from a strengths-based standpoint that alongside the characteristics widely known to be helpful for increasing the therapeutic alliance and facilitating change (i.e., warmth, genuineness, empathy) should be a genuine overarching level of therapeutic respect (Serran et al., 2003). Firesetting behaviour can often elicit negative stereotypes and connotations (e.g., "weird Pete down the road"; see Amos, 2019), so it is critical that the therapist leading treatment demonstrates genuine respect for their treatment members. A strengths-based approach promotes respectful ways of engaging with treatment members through the use of considerate language (i.e., asking how an individual would prefer to be addressed) and avoidance of pathologizing labels such as "firesetter" or "arsonist" that view individuals via an offending lens (see Willis, 2018). Strengths-based approaches also acknowledge and respect a person's competencies and talents to improve their overall life quality.

Developing a Strong and Cohesive Group

The development of a strong and cohesive group, as noted earlier, is highly dependent upon providing individuals with a safe and supportive group environment. Displaying therapist features known to be helpful for increasing the therapeutic alliance is important in this endeavour (i.e., warmth, genuineness, empathy; see Marshall & Burton, 2010 or Marshall et al., 2013) as is encouraging group members to treat each other in a similarly respectful manner. During the initial stages of our FIPP or FIP-MO treatment, we concentrate fully on the process of ensuring that individuals feel safe and supported to attend the group. For example, apart from asking individuals about their hopes and fears regarding the group, we pay little attention to the concept of firesetting. Instead, we focus on getting to know one another in a relaxed and positive manner. For example, we ask individuals to tell us about their strengths, invite the group to generate rules around group behaviour to make everyone feel comfortable, and encourage individuals to highlight something positive they have noticed about one another.

Therapists are expected to lead the group and engage in behaviours known to be helpful for facilitating behaviour change (i.e., be directive and reward shifts in behaviour effectively; Marshall et al., 2002, 2003). We also encourage an egalitarian atmosphere in which therapists "check in" alongside group members about their week, sit together with group members during their coffee break, and engage in group tasks asked of group members where appropriate. "Check ins" and engagement in group tasks need not be overly disclosive. A therapist can model appropriate challenges in their life without becoming overly descriptive (e.g., "I met an old friend last week, and it made me realise how little time I have spent staying connected with supportive friends"). Research supports the idea that therapists should represent models of coping rather than models of mastery via appropriate and deliberately used disclosures (see Henretty & Levitt, 2010; Henretty et al., 2014; Hill et al., 2018; Serran et al., 2003). In fact, skilled self-disclosure and flexibility in treatment represent important therapist features (Marshall & Burton, 2010; Marshall et al., 2013; Serran et al., 2003).

Being flexible regarding the needs of individual group members is a vital therapist skill. To develop group cohesion, individuals need to develop some sense of a shared emotional experience (see Rimé, 2007, 2009). An emotionally sensitive therapist will detect a group member's emotional state and decide whether the group theme requires shifting to support that particular group member. For example, an individual who "checks in" at the beginning of a group to say that they have received news that their child is to be adopted will require support and empathy from both the therapist and other group members. A skilled therapist will provide the group with the necessary support and space to share appropriate emotional experiences of loss and support the group member in question rather than moving forward prematurely with a planned activity. Such shared emotional experiences are critical for the development of group bonds and social solidarity (Rimé, 2007).

Using Group Member Strengths Effectively

All groups have members characterised by varying strengths. These strengths are likely to have become apparent during the assessment period when the assessor asks individuals about their individual talents, examines the individual's unique pattern of psychological strengths and vulnerabilities in relation to their offending, and gathers information about the individual's previous experience of groups (see Chapter 6). Typically, we have found that individuals who have received previous treatment or psychological support that they perceived to be useful tend to approach firesetting work positively. For this reason, these people tend to be positive role models for others during the early stages of the group and can be called upon first in group discussions. For example, in discussions around expectations in relation to the group, these individuals tend to exhibit appropriate hopes (e.g., "I hope to understand more about why I set fires") and realistic fears (e.g., "I'm worried about getting to the end of the group and not feeling any different"). Others, who are perhaps more apprehensive about joining the group, should be allowed to watch pro-treatment group members speak before being encouraged to express their views. Similarly, when a particularly tricky group exercise is planned (e.g., presenting information on the lead up to the firesetting), it is always worth thinking about who would be best to present first. Individuals who are open and reflective about their lives in the lead up to their offences represent effective and appropriate role models for the group. As the group continues, however, it is important not to continuously rely on particular group members to begin discussions or presentations. Doing so could elicit negative feelings that group members are being favoured in some way and could block other group members from opportunities to strengthen appropriate displays of reflection and emotional expression.

As the group continues, therapists should remain mindful of the strengths and competencies held by group members and of how these strengths can be used to benefit other group members. For example, a grievance trajectory individual may be assisted in discovering useful anger regulation techniques from members of the group exhibiting newly discovered or pre-existing strengths in this area. Furthermore, a therapist looking for a group member to engage in appropriate peer challenge of a particularly vulnerable individual might choose to elicit the views of an individual who holds strengths in communication skills.

Denial

As noted earlier, denial is relatively common amongst individuals who have offended (see Dealey, 2018), and many firesetting groups will have at least one individual attending who denies some or all of their firesetting. At the time of writing this book, we are unaware of any research examining the relationship between denial and firesetting reoffending. Research conducted in the area of sexual offending, however, suggests that denial does not typically increase reoffending (Harkins et al., 2015; Ware & Blagden, 2020), and denial is viewed as being an adaptive self-protection mechanism that should not be the focus of challenge or treatment focus (Harkins et al., 2015; Marshall et al., 2001; Ware & Marshall, 2008; Ware et al., 2020).

In our practice, we have approached the treatment of firesetting similarly. Akin with Marshall et al. (2001, 2005) and Ware and Marshall (2008), we find that individuals who have set fires vary hugely regarding the elements of their firesetting that they recall, accept, or feel responsible for. In situations when an individual denies having set a fire altogether, we set to work examining how it is they came to be accused of a firesetting offence. Typically, this highlights areas of treatment need likely to be important for reducing the risks associated with firesetting (e.g., inappropriate fire interest, offence-supportive attitudes, emotional regulation issues, communication issues; Gannon & Lockerbie, 2014; Gannon et al., 2012, 2015; Tyler et al., 2018). For example, a group member might tell the group that they were accused of setting fire to their employer's business because they were fired for clocking in late consistently. This group member might also state that their employer "deserved" what happened to them since everyone disliked this employer, so any employee could have set the fire. This level of information will be enough for the group to explore emotional regulation issues surrounding poor work performance (e.g., Why was the group member late? Were they unable to cope?) as well as offence-supportive attitudes (e.g., Is it okay for people to take the law into their own hands?). In other groups, we have had individuals telling us that they were accused of firesetting because others knew of their interest in fire, so they were an "easy target." This has allowed us to examine the concept of inappropriate fire interest with them in detail despite their complete denial of the offence. We have experienced group members who began the treatment in complete denial decide—without any prompting—that they need to inform the group that they *did* actually set the fire they were accused of. Typically, this has occurred in the context of developing group cohesiveness when individuals have seen other group members' openness and have seemingly been prompted to reciprocate.

Similarly, when individuals state that they are unable to recall the offence or events surrounding their offence in any way, we do not pressure them to recall these events or challenge their recall (cf. Marshall et al., 2005). Instead, we tell them that individuals often have problems remembering the exact details around an unusual, significant, or distressing event. We reassure them that, in time, details may become more accessible to them as they progress through the group, and we positively reinforce any information that they discuss in the lead up to the offence as the group progresses. In fact, early on in the group, when an individual minimises their involvement or excuses their involvement in the firesetting, we take an approach in line with Maruna and Mann (2006). That is, we view such excuses as functional attempts to reduce stress and maintain shame and self-esteem, and we do not challenge them (see also Farmer et al., 2016). Instead, we listen carefully to what is being said within these excuses and use this information to provide us with valuable information as to what was happening in the individual's life at the time of the firesetting offence (see Maruna & Mann, 2006). For example, an individual who states that they "only" did it because they were high on drugs is providing valuable information about how they were functioning in the lead up to their offence.

Inappropriate Group Behaviour

It is not unusual for offence-related treatment groups to face challenges associated with inappropriate behaviour occurring within the group. Such behaviours can range from the relatively minor (e.g., someone looking disinterested when a group member is talking) to more serious incidents (e.g., a physical altercation in the group). Treatment groups for firesetting are no different from other offence-related treatment groups in this respect. We have facilitated groups in which members have fallen asleep, taken over group sessions with excessive talk about their own life circumstances, shown disinterest in others' life stories, made rude remarks to others, laughed inappropriately at another group member's distress, thrown physical objects when angry, or made inappropriate sexual comments towards the therapist. In terms of fire-specific themes, we have witnessed animated group members jump up and bring out lit lighters during discussions, shout fire-supportive statements, or run around the room when viewing fire stimuli.

We view such challenges as necessary for developing emotional communication skills, reflective insight, and overall group cohesiveness (see Marshall et al., 2011; Serran, 2017 for discussions around comprehensive emotionally focused therapy). In our view, every element of a group that appears to "go wrong" is an opportunity for the development and learning of all parties (i.e., both group members and therapists). When a group member falls asleep, it may warrant enquiry. Has something happened to interrupt that person's sleep? Is it a side effect of medication? Or is the individual insufficiently connected with the group and its purpose? Typically, making an enquiry about something seemingly innocuous such as falling asleep in group can elicit highly meaningful information (e.g., "I felt at risk in my cell last night and didn't sleep," "I'm really fed up with the side effects of this medication," "I don't know why I am doing this group. I'm angry that I've been asked to attend it"). Even a group altercation can bring about genuine reflection on key issues and further strengthen group cohesion. For example, in one of our groups, an individual best described by the antisocial trajectory of the M-TTAF made some well-intended challenges of an individual best described by the emotionally expressive M-TTAF trajectory. Although the challenge made by the antisocial trajectory individual was not intended to be critical, it was clumsy and led to the emotionally expressive individual becoming overwhelmed with frustration and anger, paralleling how he had felt around the time of his firesetting. This group member got so upset that he ran out of the group room and kicked over a chair in frustration as he left. As he sat in the corridor upset and shaking, one of the therapists was able to guide him to deescalate his emotion with simple techniques. Whilst this was occurring, the remaining group talked about what had happened. Using feedback from peers, the antisocial individual was able to reflect on his questioning style, which he concluded had been too aggressive ("My question was too strong"). When the emotionally expressive individual returned to the group, both individuals were supported and encouraged to reflect on what had happened in the room and how they had reacted. The emotionally expressive individual spontaneously apologised to the group for his outburst and explained that he found it hard to accept feedback. Following some support from the therapist, it transpired that this group member's father had criticised him constantly as a child. He stated that he wanted to work on this aspect of himself in the group. The group confirmed that it had been helpful to see this behaviour directly to support this particular group member. The antisocial individual apologised for the aggressiveness of his challenge and reflected on how he could deliver feedback more sensitively.

In vivo emotional expression is extremely important for bringing about change in therapeutic groups (Gannon & Ward, 2017; Peluso & Freund, 2018; Serran, 2017). A group that avoids emotional expression tends to operate at the propositional or rational verbal level (Teasdale, 1997; Teasdale & Barnard, 1993) and will simply increase academic knowledge around a topic in the absence of meaningful self-connection (see Gannon & Ward, 2017). To connect more deeply with materials and "feel" something to be true, non-verbal levels of implicational processing or emotional processing (Teasdale, 1997; Teasdale & Barnard, 1993) must be targeted. A variety of therapeutic techniques may be used to achieve experiential change. However, these strategies all tend to require some experience of in vivo emotional activation (see Gannon & Ward, 2017). The most naturalistic, perhaps, would involve the therapist assisting a group member to cognitively examine a strong episode of affective experience (see Peluso & Freund, 2018). In the example mentioned earlier of the strong challenge that went wrong, this involved the emotionally expressive individual cognitively evaluating the event that triggered his affective reaction and bringing meaning to this event (Peluso & Freund, 2018; Teasdale, 1999).

Skilfully working with emotional activation as it occurs in the group is vital for bringing about effective emotional and cognitive change. For example, in one of our groups, an individual with a high level of inappropriate interest in fire became animated during a discussion around fire spread. He maintained that when victims died or were hurt in blazes, it was generally their fault for not getting out in time since speed of fire spread was exaggerated. He was shown a simple film of a real front room fire starting on a chair and was asked to predict how long it would take for the entire sitting room to be ablaze. The therapist logged his predictions and asked the rest of the group to also make predictions and partake in the exercise. Once the predictions had been logged, the film was left to run, and the group member in question was able to experience for himself that his predictions were considerably slower than the fire spread that he was himself timing. This is an example of an in vivo *behavioural experiment* designed to test the accuracy of a group member's beliefs (see Bennett-Levy et al., 2004). Behavioural experiments work well in vivo but can also be planned to specifically test offence-supportive beliefs or indeed other beliefs that may be impacting on the person's life or ability to engage in therapy. For example, a group member experiencing paranoia in one of our FIP-MO groups was convinced that others would be able to hear him talking in the group from outside the room. In fact, he felt he could not continue attending the group because of this. One of the therapists took this individual out of the group room into the surrounding corridors so that he could experience for himself what could or could not be heard from the corridors. He learnt from this experience that although some conversational noise could be heard in the corridor immediately outside the group room, he could not inform the group as a whole what they had been talking about when he returned. Although he needed to engage in this exercise repeatedly, this individual still attended the group and completed it successfully.

A Note on Collaborative Working and Modularisation

An important part of strengths-based treatment is its collaborative nature. Thus, a key emphasis of treatment should be on the group aiding the individual to piece together and understand how his or her firesetting came about. Together, the group can also help the individual to develop the necessary skills to lead a pro-social life and identify any problematic areas of life functioning associated with firesetting behaviour were these to occur in the future. Supporting an individual to "discover" what a good life might look like for them is an important job and therapists should be mindful of what will be realistic for each individual. For example, for an individual who holds an inappropriate interest in fire and who wants to gain mastery experiences through work, working in a fireworks factory may not be the most realistic occupational choice.

Within the FIPP and the FIP-MO, information to be covered by the group is presented as a series of "modules" which pinpoint particular areas to be explored so that group members can further understand their behaviour and develop the skills to lead a pro-social life. Key modules, for example, include fire interest or preference, communication and relationships, and exploring offence patterns. However, each of the therapist manuals accompanying the FIPP and FIP-MO are semi-structured to enhance therapist flexibility (which is an important therapeutic skill; see Marshall & Burton, 2010; Marshall et al., 2013; Serran et al., 2003). Thus, although particular elements of human functioning are separated out throughout the programme for the sake of clarity, akin with Rockwood's programme for individuals who have sexually offended (Marshall et al., 2001; W. Marshall, personal communication, May, 2008; Serran, 2017), we encourage therapists to work with any aspect of relevance as it crops up on the programme. For example, a particular group member might come to the group with a very pertinent issue (e.g., relationship loss) which necessitates work around this area, or an individual might mention their fire interest very early in the group before this module is planned to be covered in depth. In these instances, it is important that therapists are mindful of an opportunity to be flexible and feel comfortable orchestrating group work adaptably. This approach is likely to assist individuals in making valuable connections between modules as well as meaningful change (see also Serran, 2017).

Considerations for Working with Specific Populations

Women

Research suggests several common themes among female and male individuals who set deliberate fires (e.g., inappropriate fire interest, coping issues, Alleyne et al., 2016; Ó Ciardha et al., 2015b). Nevertheless, these needs are likely to manifest themselves differently as a result of gender. Although the M-TTAF hypothesises that women are more or less likely to occupy particular trajectories of the M-TTAF Tier 2 (i.e., more likely to be emotionally expressive and less likely to be antisocial), research has not yet determined exactly how women differ from men in the trajectories that lead them towards deliberate firesetting. Thus, when working with women, we tend to take a generally gender-informed approach.[1]

Our approach takes into account the high rates of trauma reported for women (Green et al., 2005; Holbrook et al., 2002), as well as their relational style (see Blanchette & Brown, 2006; O'Meara et al., 2020). Within the FIPP and the FIP-MO, trauma is viewed as an important experience that can help to explain relational patterns and ways of functioning that may have fostered firesetting. Of particular importance when assessing whether a woman should come onto a firesetting group is whether that individual holds the basic skills to self-soothe or cope with distressing emotions such as shame were they to occur in the group. If pre-existing trauma is high, then it may well be necessary to resolve that trauma prior to group work (see Trauma). Otherwise, preparatory work on how to self-soothe (e.g., compassionate mind work; Gilbert, 2011; Gilbert & Procter, 2006 or DBT; Linehan, 2015) can be extremely beneficial.

We have found that once engaged in treatment, women's relational styles are very different to men's. In line with Miller's (1976) conceptualisation of gender differences in relational theory, we find that relational connection is often extremely important to women (see also Bloom et al., 2002). Not only are blockages in these connections apparent when tracking women's lives in the lead up to their offending, but their conception of a good life also tends to be heavily centred on the experience of relatedness. Thus, women are likely to especially benefit from work examining the concepts of attachments, relational styles, and healthy relationships. This preference for connections is often seen in groups, where women will seek out close (and sometimes exclusive) bonds with other group members. Care needs to be taken when this occurs to ensure that all group members feel part of the group and that cliques do not form.

In terms of communication styles, our experience of all-female groups tends to support the gender communication differences reported by De Lance (1995). Women appear more able to disclose the past events that led to their firesetting; in fact, at times we have had to encourage individuals to wait before disclosing this element rather than prompt for information. We have also found that all-female groups tend to, on balance, involve more emotional expression and empathic gestures, which enable group cohesion to form relatively quickly. The biggest barrier experienced in all-female groups can be related to the relational bonds made in the group. Occasionally, members of all-female groups fall out with each other due to issues that have occurred on the wing or ward. This, however, presents therapists with a unique in vivo opportunity to work with group members on their emotions, conflict de-escalation, and relationship skills.

Individuals Experiencing Mental Illness

The M-TTAF hypothesises mental illness to be a key moderator in the sequalae of firesetting behaviour. In other words, poor mental health simply exacerbates underlying vulnerabilities such that they become critical risk factors associated with deliberate firesetting (see Chapter 3). Thus, our approach to individuals experiencing mental illness is that we welcome them onto firesetting treatment (whether they are in a prison or hospital environment). The only caveat we apply concerns whether an individual is well enough to partake in treatment. Generally, for example, if we are working within the hospital setting, we ask for input on this element from the patient's multi-disciplinary team (MDT) and then conduct our own clinical assessment of this if the MDT thinks that the patient is well enough to be approached regarding treatment. Similarly, in prisons, we invite health care to input and then conduct our own clinical assessment as appropriate. Generally, if an individual is currently suicidal or actively responding to hallucinations, then we revisit them at another treatment intake later down the line to see if these features have shown improvement. For individuals who are generally stable and who are able to deal with their hallucinations effectively, we find that they are generally able to manage group treatment well. In such circumstances, we always examine the role of mental health in relation to their firesetting participation at intake (e.g., how does the individual view the role of their mental health in relation to firesetting?; how might mental health impact upon treatment participation?). Sometimes we find that incoming group members hold very simplistic views of how their firesetting was related to their mental health (e.g., "I became unwell, and that's why I set a fire"). In such cases, we work with them throughout treatment to aid their understanding of the possible links between mental health and firesetting and present them with information suggesting that mental health is not always directly related to criminal behaviour (e.g., Elbogen & Johnson, 2009). In fact, the exact function of the mental health issue should be formulated carefully since, in some cases, command hallucinations appear to exacerbate or unleash pre-existing issues (e.g., aggressiveness, inappropriate fire interest). Formulating the links carefully enables individuals to work not only on their mental health but also on the other relevant factors likely to be involved in their firesetting (i.e., critical risk factors from the M-TTAF; see Chapter 3).

Conclusions, Ways of Working, and Future Directions

In this chapter, we have examined how best to engage and work therapeutically with firesetting behaviour using strengths-based approaches. Because firesetting is such an under-studied topic, we have extrapolated from other therapeutic areas (i.e., work with individuals who have sexually offended; general psychotherapeutic research and principles) as well as our own clinical experience of running the FIPP or FIP-MO. Overall, our key messages are as follows. First, when thinking about suitable treatment candidates, therapists should view individuals across the entire spectrum of the M-TTAF trajectories as being suitable group members (including the antisocial trajectory) and should seek to set up as diverse group as possible, including diversity regarding offence denial and accountability. Second, when approaching and interacting with treatment candidates, therapists should be mindful of and equipped to deal with the stigma associated with firesetting and of the apprehension individuals are likely to display regarding group-based treatment. Trauma, in particular, is one area that therapists should seek to appraise early in the process to ensure that individuals are robust enough to tolerate treatment for their firesetting. Third, when navigating group work, therapists should seek to establish a safe and supportive atmosphere in order to foster a strong and cohesive group. Towards this aim, it is paramount that therapists display therapist features known to increase the therapeutic alliance (e.g., warmth, genuineness, empathy; Marshall & Burton, 2010; Marshall et al., 2013). Fourth, therapists should concentrate on and elicit the strengths of group members to examine how they can live an offence-free life as well as how these strengths might benefit other group members. Fifth, therapists should view difficult discussions and behaviour in the group as an "opportunity" rather than a failure of treatment. In vivo emotional expression is critical for positive outcomes, and therapists should engage with this process and aid their clients to attach cognitive meaning to any expressed emotion (Peluso & Freund, 2018). Finally, therapists should be flexible and work with aspects of problematic functioning as it occurs in the group rather than artificially examining particular psychological components within specific modules (Serran, 2017).

Our knowledge of how to engage and work with individuals who have set fires is very much in the developmental stages. For example, we need to know more about how group diversity on the various M-TTAF trajectories impacts treatment outcome and whether denial has a relationship with fire reoffending similar to that documented in the sexual offence literature. Further work is also needed to aid our understanding regarding group cohesiveness and how best to generate and maintain it within groups targeting firesetting behaviour. Until then practitioners working with individuals who have set fires should consult the general literature regarding strengths-based treatment and effective group process and therapist features.

Note

1 Gender-informed interventions are not simply more palatable to women; they are also associated with reductions in reoffending (see Gobeil et al.'s, 2016 meta-analysis).

8

What Next? The Future of Firesetting Research and Practice

In this closing chapter, we draw on key themes from earlier chapters to consider the future of research and practice in the area of adult deliberate firesetting. In particular, we examine key developments in theory, assessment, and treatment. We also identify key trends in research, developments that have been made, and research priorities we view as paramount for future progression and innovation in this area. We hope readers will find this chapter helpful for thinking about what to prioritise when planning and designing research, developing theory, or providing interventions in the area of deliberate firesetting.

Developments and Priorities

Theoretical Understanding

There is no doubt that professionals know significantly more about the aetiology of adult deliberate firesetting than was known just a few decades ago. In the 1970s and early 1980s, for example, there was a complete absence of multi-factorial explanations of deliberate firesetting. Instead, the field was dominated by simple typological approaches that categorised individuals into subtypes based on their offence characteristics or key motives underpinning their deliberate firesetting (Bradford, 1982; Inciardi, 1970; Levin, 1976; Scott, 1974). During these decades, psychoanalytical theory (Freud, 1932) and social learning theory (Bandura, 1976) were the only prominent single-factor explanations of deliberate firesetting. Whilst psychoanalytical theory has not stood the test of time and empirical scrutiny (Ó Ciardha, 2015c; Quinsey et al., 1989), social learning theory has received some empirical support as being an important aetiological factor underpinning deliberate firesetting (e.g., Barnoux et al., 2015) and has remained an appealing avenue of explanation for both researchers and practitioners (Gannon et al., 2012; see Chapter 3).

In the 1980s and 1990s, two pioneering figures—Kenneth Fineman (1980, 1995) and Howard Jackson (1994, Jackson et al., 1987)—independently began developing professional understanding of deliberately set fires through generating multi-factorial explanations. Jackson and his colleagues (1987) favoured a clinical functional analysis approach with strong social learning theory underpinnings and Fineman (1980, 1995) a dynamic behavioural approach. Both approaches were highly influential since they were able to explain, for the first time, how a host of social, environmental, and psychological factors culminated to explain deliberate firesetting. These theories also viewed fire interest as being important, if not central, to deliberate firesetting behaviour, enabling clinicians to formulate this seemingly mysterious behaviour in a theoretically informed manner for the very first time. However, this focus meant that only individuals who held an expressed interest in fire could be formulated competently. What was missing from the academic literature was information to aid clinicians who were dealing with clients who had set fires and yet appeared to hold appropriate levels of fire interest (e.g., fires set to cover up another crime or to falsely claim insurance money).

Jackson (1994; Jackson et al., 1987) and Fineman's (1980, 1995) theories were the only multi-factorial theories available to describe deliberate firesetting for more than two decades. In 2012, however, following the publication of a review of the state of the literature by Gannon and Pina (2010), the Multi-Trajectory Theory of Adult Firesetting (M-TTAF; Gannon et al., 2012; see Chapter 3) was developed. The M-TTAF adopted the concept of theory knitting (Kalmar & Sternberg, 1988) to knit together the strengths of Jackson's functional analysis theory (Jackson, 1994; Jackson et al., 1987) and Fineman's dynamic behavioural theory (1980, 1995) with contemporary research and clinical information around deliberate firesetting. In a significant departure from previous multi-factorial theories of firesetting, the M-TTAF attempted to explain adult deliberate firesetting that occurred both in the presence or *absence* of inappropriate fire interest. The latter firesetting was explained through introducing the concept of an inappropriate fire script. Inappropriate fire scripts— or cognitions regarding how fire should be used and in what contexts—were hypothesised to develop as a result of social learning experiences and to guide an individual's choice to misuse fire. For example, an individual who, as a child, witnessed an older brother misusing fire to scare others while avoiding direct confrontation might learn to use fire as a way of indirectly aggressing against others (an example of the aggression-fire fusion script; Gannon et al., 2012). As discussed in Chapter 3, while no theory is perfect, the M-TTAF holds a number of strengths relative to its predecessors. Most notable perhaps is that it accounts for both male and female perpetrators of firesetting as well as varying mental health presentations. It also describes particular subtypes or trajectories of adults who set deliberate fires and provides a description of their likely clinical features which is appealing for treatment providers. Yet while the M-TTAF has received some empirical support for these subtypes from researchers independent to the model developers (see Campbell, 2016; Dalhuisen et al., 2017; Long et al., 2014; Nanayakkara et al., 2020a), further work is needed not only to substantiate the subtypes but also to flesh out particular aspects of the model. For example, although the M-TTAF predicts that culture is an important factor in the development of beliefs and attitudes around fire, we know almost nothing about the role that culture plays in facilitating or protecting individuals from engaging in fire misuse. Furthermore, research needs to be structured around many of the M-TTAF's factors and its proposed aetiological mechanisms to substantiate or revise the M-TTAF or provide competing theories to advance the adult firesetting field. Similar to Dickens et al. (2016), we believe that to push the field forward, researchers must *prospectively* operationalise their variables to test elements of the M-TTAF rather than using ill-fitting retrospective data to test the M-TTAF's complex trajectories. In conducting such research, professionals should also be mindful of best practice design and analysis to ensure their research meets the standards of rigour required for excellent quantitative and qualitative research (see the General Research Considerations section).

In recent years, two offence process models have been developed using grounded theory methods to describe the key events that precede and accompany deliberate firesetting (Barnoux et al., 2015; Tyler et al., 2014). These models were developed from the narratives of adults who had deliberately set fires and who were either resident in prisons (Barnoux et al., 2015; 38 males) or forensic mental health hospitals (Tyler et al., 2014; 16 men and 7 women). These models have improved our understanding of the types of experiences and events that put men at risk of firesetting. Such models can be particularly helpful for therapists and clients in the treatment context since they can highlight where in the sequence of events prior to the deliberate firesetting action decision making became intentionally or unintentionally risky. Although further validation of these models would be useful, there is also a need to generate models that specifically focus on women who have set deliberate fires to see if their chain of events differs in any meaningful way to that described by men. Furthermore, it would be particularly illuminating to generate offence process models using individuals from varying countries and contexts who have set deliberate fires (e.g., bushfire versus property fires). For example, the models generated by Barnoux et al. (2015) and Tyler et al. (2014) were developed using mainly British firesetters' narratives, which centred around setting fire to properties (e.g., houses and cars). It would be informative to generate a model that, for example, is based on the narratives of both Indigenous and non-Indigenous individuals who have set property fires and/or bushfires in Australia. This would enable therapists to inform their practice using socially, culturally, and geographically sensitive models.

Perhaps one of the biggest theoretical issues yet to be addressed in the field relates to un-apprehended firesetting. As noted in Chapter 5, the detection and clearance rates for deliberate fires are very low (e.g., 5.7% for England and Wales between 2015 and 2016; Arson Prevention Forum, 2017). In other words, the majority of people responsible for setting deliberate fires remain un-apprehended. Although research is beginning to make some headway in describing the basic characteristics of these individuals and their motivations for firesetting (see Barrowcliffe, 2017; Barrowcliffe & Gannon, 2015, 2016; Blanco et al., 2010; Gannon & Barrowcliffe, 2012; Hoertel et al., 2011; Vaughn et al., 2010, Chapter 5), none of the theoretical developments described in this book account for these individuals. Consequently, a particularly pressing need is to develop new theories—or perhaps amend existing ones—to provide an aetiological explanation of deliberate firesetting associated with the largest group of adults who engage in this behaviour (i.e., un-apprehended individuals). Developing a multi-factorial theory will require some significant expansion of existing research efforts on this topic. We still know little about these individuals or how they evade apprehension. In the short term, it would make sense to develop offence process models on this topic to understand more about the sequence of events leading up to and surrounding an un-apprehended firesetting event, as well as to identify potential points in the aetiological pathway for prevention. Clearly, however, researchers will need to be resourceful in planning their approach and recruitment of such participants given that their deliberate firesetting has not been formally recognised by the authorities.

Assessment

Some progress has been made in the past decade or two with developing measures to examine fire-related constructs such as fire interest and fire normalisation (see Gannon & Barrowcliffe, 2012; Gannon et al., in preparation; Murphy & Clare, 1996; Ó Ciardha et al., 2015c). For many years, the Fire Interest Rating Scale and the Fire-setting Assessment Schedule (Murphy & Clare, 1996) were the only widely available measures that could be used to assess fire interest and the events, feelings, and cognitions associated with firesetting, respectively. Both were originally developed for use with individuals with intellectual disabilities, although it was not long before they were being used with adults more generally in the absence of competing assessments. Fire interest is perhaps one of the key variables that professionals are most keen to explore when assessing an individual who has set a fire or fires. The keen focus on this element appears to be sensible given the research we have explored in this book showing that holding an inappropriate interest or fascination with fire is a key predictor for both firesetting onset and repetition (Kolko & Kazdin, 1992; McCarty & McMahon, 2005; Rice & Harris, 1996; Tyler et al., 2015). Historically, however, a key problem for professionals examining fire interest using the Fire Interest Rating Scale (Murphy & Clare, 1996) has been that there was no guidance on what might constitute a concerning response or set of responses. In the absence of any cut-off scores or guiding norms, this meant that professionals had to use their own clinical judgment to highlight potentially problematic responses. A decade later, Ó Ciardha and colleagues (Ó Ciardha et al., 2015b, 2015c) combined the Fire Interest Rating Scale (Murphy & Clare, 1996) with an unpublished measure of fire attitudes (the Fire Attitude Scale; Muckley, 1997) and an unpublished measure of identification with fire (the Identification with Fire Questionnaire; Gannon et al., 2011). Using a sample of imprisoned men who had either set a fire or not, Ó Ciardha and his colleagues factor analysed the items across these measures and identified four final factors (or subscales) that differentiated firesetting and non-firesetting individuals named the Four Factor Fire Scale (FFFS). These subscales were labelled identification with fire, serious fire interest, fire safety awareness, and normalisation of firesetting. In their 2016 journal article, Ó Ciardha et al. calculated clinical cut off scores for varying client groups (i.e., male and female prisoners or forensic mental health patients) to provide practitioners with information to contextualise client scores relative to these samples. While this approach has encouraged practitioners to move away from adopting a purely clinical judgement-based approach to the interpretation of questionnaire measures, the samples that the FFFS was based on were UK-based, selective, and relatively small. One of the notable issues with the FFFS is that because it is based on older measures, it does not reflect latest theoretical thinking regarding the fire-related factors underpinning firesetting (e.g., inappropriate fire scripts). A further limitation is that the concepts measured by the FFFS were developed solely from the literature and findings established with apprehended individuals who have set fires.

Few assessment measures have been developed and tested using un-apprehended individuals who report having set fires (see the Fire Setting and Fire Proclivity Scales; Barrowcliffe & Gannon, 2015, 2016; Gannon & Barrowcliffe, 2012), and such measures have not generally been used with apprehended samples. More recently, Gannon et al. (in preparation) combined the FFFS items and items from the fire interest subscale of the Fire Setting Scale (Gannon & Barrowcliffe, 2012) with 117 new items generated to reflect theoretical developments in adult deliberate firesetting (i.e., Butler & Gannon's, [2015] scripts).

In a two-part study, Gannon et al. first tested the full batch of items with 1,402 community participants, just under 10% of whom self-reported having set a deliberate fire that they had never been apprehended for. Gannon and colleagues' exploratory and confirmatory factor analyses suggested a strong final questionnaire comprised of eight subscales. Four of these (firesetting as normal, identification with fire, fire safety, and pathological fire interest) reflected concepts measured by the FFFS, and one (fire interest) reflected the concept of more basic fire interest incorporated in a previous version of the FFFS (see Ó Ciardha et al., 2015b). The remaining three subscales measured the new and theoretically meaningful concepts of coping using fire (i.e., a fire coping script), fire is a powerful messenger (i.e., the fire is a powerful messenger script), and fascination with fire paraphernalia (i.e., being interested in the activity, personnel, and equipment associated with fire). The final questionnaire was then validated with 101 incarcerated men (approximately half of whom had set deliberate fires) and male community members. This final questionnaire—particularly the total score—demonstrated moderate to large effects when associated with various firesetting criteria (e.g., convictions for firesetting, any lifetime firesetting).

Although the initial findings regarding the Firesetting Questionnaire appear positive, future large-scale research validating the measure with various populations (e.g., mental health patients, women who have set deliberate fires) is required. Additionally, there are no guarantees that this measure would be valid for use globally or cross-culturally. Clearly, future work on firesetting assessment measures needs to prioritise this issue and employ cultural consultants to partake in the adaptation of existing measures or development of new measures for cultural groups that have not been represented appropriately in the literature so far.

To date, all of the assessments designed to examine fire-related constructs such as inappropriate fire interest have tended to rely on traditional questionnaire or self-report measures. Recently, researchers have begun to employ cognitive-experimental methods that attempt to assess the characteristics of individuals who have set fires without relying on conscious self-report avenues (Barrowcliffe et al., 2019; Butler & Gannon, 2021; Sambrooks, 2021). For example, Sambrooks (2021) has been comparing the measurement of fire interest using more traditional methods (i.e., asking participants to imagine a firesetting scene) with a tailor made virtual reality immersive environment involving fire to see if the immersive fire environment prompts naturalistic fire cognition and affect associated with fire interest. The outcomes of this research are yet to be analysed and reported. However, this study illustrates that there is much potential for innovation and exploration in the area of assessment protocols for individuals who have set deliberate fires.

Unfortunately, as outlined in Chapter 4, relative to other fields of criminal behaviour, little progress has been made over the past few decades on the issue of risk assessment for individuals who have set deliberate fires. In fact, our scholarly understanding of criminal firesetting risk prediction still remains decades behind that of other criminal behaviours (see Dickens et al., 2016). For example, in the area of general violence, over 200 structured risk assessments have been developed and are being used by professionals to predict and manage violence across the globe (Singh et al., 2014). Yet there is not a single validated risk assessment tool worldwide to assist professionals with the serious issue of adult deliberate firesetting. This is despite recent meta-analytic evidence suggesting that as many as one in five individuals with a previous firesetting offence go on to re-offend using fire (Sambrooks et al., 2021). A small number of both published and unpublished tools have been designed by professionals (Logan et al., 2010; Long et al., 2013; Taylor & Thorne, 2013, 2019). However, these measures do not generally reflect latest theoretical developments in the field (e.g., the concept of inappropriate fire scripts) and remain unvalidated. Until a validated tool exists, we have advocated that professionals tasked with firesetting risk assessment adopt a theoretically informed structured professional judgement approach using the M-TTAF (Gannon et al., 2012) as the guiding template (see Chapter 4).

The key problem underpinning the lack of a validated risk assessment tool stems from a basic lack of research in areas that would support the development of such a tool. For example, although we know a little about the static risk predictors of firesetting, very few studies measure the potential dynamic risk factors of individuals who have set fires and track these individuals to examine which of these factors predict future repeat firesetting. Prospective studies are likely to be particularly powerful for making gains in this area of research (see Rice & Harris, 1996 for a good example). However, such studies tend to be time consuming and costly, necessitating research funding. Nevertheless, such studies will be crucial for developing the evidence base in this important area.

A further associated issue underpinning the lack of validated risk assessment tools to date relates to the complexity of firesetting as a behaviour relative to other types of offending. A key factor in this respect is offence outcome severity. During a general physical assault, a perpetrator can exert relative control over the outcome. When fire is used, however, a whole host of physical and environmental factors come into play that impact the physical properties of the fire (e.g., fuel type, wind speed) and its associated outcomes. One small-scale study (Dickens et al., 2009) was unable to link psychological intent to endanger life with firesetting outcome severity yet suggested that fires with the most severe human and economic outcomes were more likely to have been set by individuals who experienced tension and excitement at the time of the fire and who used accelerants and multiple ignition points. Ultimately, we need to determine which cluster of psychological and environmental factors offers the best predictive capability for determining firesetting severity in terms of loss of life and economic cost. Determining this will undoubtedly bring the firesetting field to a new frontier in terms of risk assessment approaches. However, this can only occur if professionals engage in best practice design and analysis (see the General Research Considerations section).

Treatment

Globally, the past few decades have been characterised by very little emphasis on specialist interventions for adults who set deliberate fires (see Chapter 6). It is unclear why such little effort has been made in this area when treatments for other offence types such as sexual offending have proliferated. Gannon and Pina (2010) concluded that professionals had taken the "intuitively appealing" (p. 233) route of assuming that individuals who set deliberate fires—with their varied offence histories—needed non-specialist programmes typically offered to the general offending population (e.g., social skills or assertiveness programmes). Yet theory and research had suggested, for some time, that adults who set deliberate fires hold fire-specific cognition and affect that play a significant role in firesetting behaviour (Gannon et al., 2013; Jackson et al., 1987; Murphy & Clare, 1996).

In the 1990s and 2000s, some professionals developed pioneering in-house treatment specifically focusing on reducing deliberate firesetting (e.g., Hall, 1995; Swaffer et al., 2001; Taylor et al., 2002; see Chapter 6). However, standardised treatment for this population only really began in the 2010s. At this point, two specialist cognitive behavioural therapy interventions began in the UK: The Firesetting Intervention Programme for Prisoners (FIPP; Gannon, 2012, 2017) and The Firesetting Intervention Programme for Mentally Disordered Offenders (FIP-MO; Gannon & Lockerbie, 2011, 2012, 2014, 2017) and one in Australia, the Australian Centre for Arson Research and Treatment Firesetter Treatment Programme (ACART; Fritzon et al., 2013). As noted in Chapter 6, all of these programmes are flexible, strengths-based programmes that utilise broad correctional rehabilitation theories (i.e., the Risk Need Responsivity Model, Bonta & Andrews, 2017; and the Good Lives Model; Ward et al., 2007) and are underpinned by contemporary firesetting theory (i.e., the M-TTAF; Gannon et al., 2012). At the time of writing, the FIPP and FIP-MO programmes are being delivered across the UK, Australia, North America, Europe, and select parts of Asia, and the ACART is being delivered in Australia.

Despite the existence of these standardised programmes designed specifically to target adult firesetting, the field of firesetting is decades behind that of other offending fields in terms of treatment knowledge. For example, professionals (e.g., Alexander et al., 2015; Chester et al., 2018) have highlighted an overrepresentation of arson convictions amongst long-stay patients in UK forensic mental health settings. This overrepresentation has been attributed to a lack of available interventions for this group, which has had an impact upon the discharge pathway (Völlm et al., 2018). Because of the paucity of research examining dynamic risk factors, professionals designing treatment have, in effect, had to make assumptions about the possible criminogenic needs to be targeted within these programmes. Determining the effectiveness of these contemporary programmes is vital for the field and is highly dependent upon best practice evaluation design that involves recidivism outcomes. All evaluations of the current available standardised treatment programmes suggest some improvement in characteristics associated with firesetting behaviour post-treatment (Fritzon et al., 2022; Gannon et al., 2015; Tyler et al., 2018), with two evaluations each incorporating a reasonably similar group of untreated individuals for comparison (Gannon et al., 2015; Tyler et al., 2018). However, to our knowledge, only the FIPP evaluation has incorporated an ongoing project that collects recidivism data for both treatment and comparison participants. At present, 7 years of follow-up data are available, the findings of which are due to be reported in the near future.

In other fields of offending behaviour (e.g., sexual offending), significant issues appear to have arisen when recidivism data associated with treatment have not been reported in a timely manner (see Brown & Ross, 2020; Mews et al., 2017). Thus, it is of paramount importance that any firesetting intervention or treatment implemented incorporates a behavioural follow-up that is communicated to the professional community in a timely manner. Furthermore, it would be ill-advised to design studies that provide such data for a treatment group without the addition of a well-matched comparison group. At this stage in developing treatment for adults who have set deliberate fires, reporting data in the absence of a well-matched comparison group could lead the field down a practice dead-end or, worse still, result in treatment that increases firesetting risk.

Thus, in our view, researchers and practitioners seeking to add value to the evaluation of firesetting treatment and intervention should seek to (1) ensure that in addition to the treatment group, they employ a group of similar individuals who are treatment eligible who either do not receive treatment or receive alternative treatment; (2) employ validated pre- and post-treatment measures to examine characteristics likely to be associated with firesetting risk and measure these across both treatment and comparison groups; and (3) integrate some type of behavioural long-term follow-up to evaluate whether the intervention or treatment is having the intended impact of reducing firesetting behaviours or behaviours likely to indicate firesetting-risk (e.g., threats to set fires). Evaluators should also seek to examine treatment non-completers to understand the characteristics of these individuals and include analyses to examine whether non-completion increases recidivism risk for some individuals as it seems to for other offending relevant programmes (Howard et al., 2018; McMurran & Theodosi, 2007). As our knowledge of firesetting risk improves, an important question will revolve around whether those at higher risk of firesetting tend to be those who are most likely to exit treatment (cf. Olver et al., 2011).

Since running standardised treatment for firesetting is a relatively recent endeavour and we have not yet gained convincing evidence of treatment effectiveness, very little is known about how professionals should work therapeutically with individuals who have set deliberate fires or which practices maximise treatment effects. Chapter 7 outlines some common challenges faced by practitioners who have recruited and therapeutically engaged participants in either the FIPP or the FIP-MO. Much of the advice presented in this chapter is based on what is known about the delivery of best practice offence-related interventions more generally (e.g., the importance of the therapeutic alliance; Marshall & Burton, 2010) paired with our clinical knowledge of adult individuals who have set deliberate fires. One area that we are commonly asked about is that of denial. To our knowledge, this topic has not yet been studied in any great depth in the area of adult perpetrated firesetting. In other areas of offending behaviour such as sexual offending, denial has not been found to be associated with increased reoffending (Harkins et al., 2015; Ware & Blagden, 2020) and has been conceptualised as a helpful self-protection strategy not to be vigorously challenged by therapists (Harkins et al., 2015; Marshall et al., 2001; Ware & Marshall, 2008; Ware et al., 2020). Although it is intuitively appealing to assume the relationship works similar to that reported in the area of sexual offending, this has not yet been empirically supported. A very useful piece of work would be to examine the relationship between denial and firesetting reoffending.

General Research Considerations

Chapter 2 highlights a number of quality issues associated with many of the research studies examining the characteristics of adults who set deliberate fires. Many of these issues stem from research design, and similar issues are noted throughout the book (e.g., for treatment evaluation design). A good number of the research studies examining firesetting were conducted many years ago, which is likely to account for some of the lack of sophistication in research design. Nevertheless, as sustained research attention grows in this area, we believe it is important to set out a research design agenda that we hope will be shared by researchers in the field to ensure that ongoing research is of a suitable quality to make valued contributions. Next, we propose what we believe are key considerations.

First, prior to any research taking place, researchers should take considerable care to plan their design and analysis strategy. One particularly effective method of doing this is to consider the pre-registration of any planned study. Pre-registration is becoming a popular practice in some psychology subdisciplines (e.g., social and experimental psychology; see van't Veer & Giner-Sorolla, 2016) but is not yet pervasive in forensic psychology. The practice of pre-registration involves the researcher specifying, in advance of their study, hypotheses to be tested, the specific design and measures to be used (including sample size specification, criteria for participant inclusion and exclusion, detailing of all relevant variables), as well as specific analyses to be conducted (Simmons et al., 2021). Most important for the field of firesetting, perhaps, is that the practice of pre-registration does not preclude exploratory study; it simply ensures that research users know which areas of the research were carefully planned (see Simmons et al., 2021). This document is time-stamped and made publicly available so that research users are assured that the outcomes are less likely to be the result of false positives generated from p-hacking (i.e., conscious or unconscious sampling or analysis decisions that increase significant findings or a more appealing patterns of results; Simmons et al., 2021). Pre-registration is a practice that can help to ensure that a study is well planned and adequately powered to find the effects hypothesised. Suitably powered studies are critical for providing the field with the well-founded evidence required to inform theoretical amendment and revision and move the field of firesetting to a new frontier.

Attention to numerous other design issues will also be helpful in ensuring that each new piece of research undertaken makes a notable difference to the field. A particularly notable problem for much early research in firesetting, as well as some contemporary research, is the lack of an adequately matched comparison group. The inclusion of such a group is crucial for drawing adequate conclusions about the key characteristics and factors associated with firesetting relative to other offending behaviour (i.e., when comparing individuals who have set deliberate fires to individuals who have offended in other ways). In such cases, it is important to consider which factors are important to match as closely as possible between the groups. For most survey studies, a good starting point would be to ensure that groups do not differ substantially on age, gender, ethnicity, or full-scale IQ. Another approach would be to match individual participants across the groups as closely as possible on such variables. For specific studies (e.g., examining risk of reoffending), it would be advisable to ensure that the participant groups do not differ substantially in terms of previous criminality. When researching individuals who have been apprehended, it can also be incredibly helpful to include a firesetting community comparison group. The inclusion of such a group is useful for indicating factors that distinguish individuals who have been identified for their firesetting from the wider community. However, it can be difficult and time consuming to make these latter comparisons since these groups are often notably different on ethnicity and socio-economic variables (see Gannon et al., in preparation). Ultimately, however, providing well-matched comparison groups pays dividends and should be included as a matter of principle unless the particular research question does not necessitate it (e.g., developing an offence process model of how firesetting occurs; Tyler et al., 2014). In our view, it is simply not defensible to publish quantitative studies on adult deliberate firesetting that do not include an adequate comparison group or an adequate estimation of study power since such studies are likely to proliferate the field with false findings that are misleading and possibly even dangerous for clinical practice.

The field of firesetting might also benefit, at this stage, from the implementation of novel research designs and methods incorporated from both psychology and other disciplines. For example, very few of the studies we have mentioned in this book have used anything other than file review or self-report methods to examine the characteristics and features associated with adults who have set deliberate fires. As we have noted earlier in this chapter, innovative research methods that aim to circumvent traditional and transparent self-report measures represent one potential avenue of research to move the field forward (e.g., Barrowcliffe et al., 2019; Sambrooks, 2021). There is also considerable room for researchers to draw upon the expertise of other disciplines (e.g., the environmental sciences) to understand more about how deliberate firesetting impacts society (e.g., what is the ecological impact of deliberate firesetting?). Incorporating new and differing perspectives has the potential to attract external research funding and move the field forward in various innovative ways.

Concluding Comments

A key theme that has arisen in this book has been that progress has been made in the past two decades on our understanding of the theory, assessment, and treatment of adult deliberate firesetting. However, a further accompanying theme has been that further research needs to be done to make significant advances, particularly in the areas of risk assessment and treatment provision and evaluation. Making these advances will be time consuming, but such work needs to be prioritised to bring the evidence base on line with other offending behaviours. We propose that practitioners and academics share their expertise and work together to plan and conduct the large-scale pieces of research needed to improve the current evidence base on adult deliberate firesetting. To move this field to the next frontier, we need to work across disciplines and settings, and we need to strive as editors, reviewers, and researchers to publish and pursue only research which is of sufficient quality to make a scientific contribution to this important field. Practitioners themselves should call for and support best practice evidence generation wherever possible, and policy makers must demand funded research programmes that enable adults who have set deliberate fires to be appropriately assessed and treated within institutions and the community. We know what needs to be done, and the time has come for all of us to work together to make this happen over the next decade.

References

Addison, C. C., Campbell-Jenkins, B. W., Sarpong, D. F., Kibler, J., Singh, M., Dubbert, P., Wilson, G., Payne, T., & Taylor, H. (2007). Psychometric evaluation of a Coping Strategies Inventory Short-Form (CSI-SF) in the Jackson heart study cohort. *International Journal of Environmental Research and Public Health, 4*(4), 289–295. https://doi.org/10.3390/ijerph200704040004

Alexander, R. T., Chester, V., Green, F. N., Gunaratna, I., & Hoare, S. (2015). Arson or fire setting in offenders with intellectual disability: Clinical characteristics, forensic histories, and treatment outcomes. *Journal of Intellectual and Developmental Disability, 40*(2), 189–197. https://doi.org/10.3109/13668250.2014.998182

All Wales Joint Arson Group (2019). *Wales arson reduction strategy (Report No. 4)*. Mid and West Wales Fire and Rescue Service, Wales, UK. https://www.mawwfire.gov.uk/media/1798/walesarsonreductionstrategy.pdf

Allender, P., Brown, G., Bailey, N., Colombo, T., Poole, H., & Saldana, A. (2005). *Prisoner resettlement and housing provision: A good practice ideas guide*. Centre for Social Justice, Coventry University. https://lemosandcrane.co.uk/resources/Prisoner_Resettlement_and_Housing_Provision.pdf

Alleyne, E., Gannon, T. A., Mozova, K., Page, T. E., & Ó Ciardha, C. (2016). Female fire-setters: Gender-associated psychological and psychopathological features. *Psychiatry, 79*(4), 364–378. https://doi.org/10.1080/00332747.2016.1185892

American Psychiatric Association (2013). Diagnostic and statistical manual of mental disorders (5th ed). Author.

Amos, O. (2019, November 14). *Australian fires: Why do people start fires during fires?* BBC News. Retrieved from https://www.bbc.co.uk/news/world-australia-50400851

Anderson, J. (2010). *Bushfire arson prevention handbook (Research in practice No. 11)*. Australian Institute of Criminology. https://www.aic.gov.au/publications/rip/rip11

Andrews, D. A., & Bonta, J. (2010). The psychology of criminal conduct (5th ed.). Matthew Bender & Company.

Andrews, D. A., Bonta, J., & Wormith, J. S. (2006). The recent past and near future of risk and/or need assessment. *Crime and Delinquency, 52*(1), 7–27. https://doi.org/10.1177/0011128705281756

Annesley, P., Davison, L., Colley, C., Gilley, L., & Thomson, L. (2017). Developing and evaluating interventions for women firesetters in high secure mental health care. *Journal of Forensic Practice, 19*(1), 59–76. https://doi.org/10.1108/JFP-12-2015-0054

Adult Deliberate Firesetting: Theory, Assessment, and Treatment, First Edition. Theresa A. Gannon, Nichola Tyler, Caoilte Ó Ciardha and Emma Alleyne.
© 2022 John Wiley & Sons Ltd. Published 2022 by John Wiley & Sons Ltd.

Anwar, S., Långström, N., Grann, M., & Fazel, S. (2011). Is arson the crime most strongly associated with psychosis? A national case-control study of arson risk in schizophrenia and other psychoses. *Schizophrenia Bulletin, 37*(3), 580–586. https://doi.org/10.1093/schbul/sbp098

Ardino, V. (2012). Offending behaviour: The role of trauma and PTSD. *European Journal of Psychotraumatology, 3*(1), 18968. https://doi.org/10.3402/ejpt.v3i0.18968

Arson Prevention Forum (2017). *State of the nation 2017*. Stop Arson UK. https://www.burgoynes.com/Media/pdf/ds2017-2297-arson-prevention-forum-booklet.pdf

Ashworth, S., Mooney, P., & Tully, R. J. (2017). A case study demonstrating the effectiveness of an adapted-DBT program upon increasing adaptive emotion management skills, with an individual diagnosed with mild learning disability and emotionally unstable personality disorder. *Journal of Forensic Psychology Research and Practice, 17*(1), 38–60. https://doi.org/10.1080/15228932.2017.1251098

Bandura, A. (1976). Self-reinforcement: Theoretical and methodological considerations. *Behaviorism, 4*(2), 135–155. Retrieved from http://www.jstor.org/stable/27758862

Barker, A. F. (1994). Arson: A review of the psychiatric literature. Oxford University Press.

Barnett, W., & Spitzer, M. (1994). Pathological fire-setting 1951-1991: A review. *Medicine, Science and the Law, 34*(1), 4–20. https://doi.org/10.1177/002580249403400103

Barnoux, M., & Gannon, T. A. (2013). A new conceptual framework for revenge firesetting. *Psychology, Crime & Law, 20*(5), 497–513. https://doi.org/10.1080/1068316X.2013.793769

Barnoux, M., Gannon, T. A., & Ó Ciardha, C. (2015). A descriptive model of the offence chain for imprisoned adult male firesetters (descriptive model of adult male firesetting). *Legal and Criminological Psychology, 20*(1), 48–67. https://doi.org/10.1111/lcrp.12071

Baron-Cohen, S., & Wheelwright, S. (2004). The empathy quotient: An investigation of adults with Asperger syndrome or high functioning autism, and normal sex differences. *Journal of Autism and Developmental Disorders, 34*(2), 163–175. https://doi.org/10.1023/B:JADD.0000022607.19833.00

Barrow, L. M., Rufo, R. A., & Arambula, S. (2014). Police and profiling in the United States: Applying theory to criminal investigations. CRC Press.

Barrowcliffe, E. R. (2017). *The prevalence and psychological characteristics on un-apprehended deliberate firesetters living in the UK* [Unpublished doctoral dissertation]. University of Kent.

Barrowcliffe, E. R., & Gannon, T. A. (2015). The characteristics of un-apprehended firesetters living in the UK community. *Psychology, Crime and Law, 21*(9), 836–853. https://doi.org/10.1080/1068316X.2015.1054385

Barrowcliffe, E. R., & Gannon, T. A. (2016). Comparing the psychological characteristics of un-apprehended firesetters and non-firesetters living in the UK. *Psychology, Crime and Law, 22*(4), 382–404. https://doi.org/10.1080/1068316X.2015.1111365

Barrowcliffe, E. R., Gannon, T. A., & Tyler, N. (2019). Measuring the cognition of firesetting individuals using explicit and implicit measures. *Psychiatry: Interpersonal and Biological Processes, 82*(4), 368–371. https://doi.org/10.1080/00332747.2019.1626201

Barrowcliffe, E. R., Tyler, N., & Gannon, T. A. (2022). Firesetting among 18-23 year old un-apprehended adults: A UK community study. *Journal of Criminological Research, Policy, and Practice*. https://doi.org/10.1108/JCRPP-06-2021-0026

Battle, J. (1992). Culture-free Self-Esteem Inventories (2nd ed.). PRO-ED.

Beck, A. T., & Beck, R. W. (1972). Screening depressed patients in family practice. *Postgraduate Medicine, 52*(6), 81–85. https://doi.org/10.1080/00325481.1972.11713319

Beech, A. R., & Fisher, D. (2011, June). *The way forward for sex offender treatment: A brain-based approach*. In *Paper Presented at the New Directions in Sex Offender Practice Conference*, University of Birmingham, Birmingham, UK.

Beech, A. R., & Hamilton-Giachritsis, C. E. (2005). Relationship between therapeutic climate and treatment outcome in group-based sexual offender treatment programs. *Sexual Abuse: A Journal of Research and Treatment, 17*(2), 127–140. https://doi.org/10.1007/s11194-005-4600-3

Bell, R., Doley, R., & Dawson, D. (2018). Developmental characteristics of firesetters: Are recidivist offenders distinctive? *Legal and Criminological Psychology, 23*(2), 163–175. https://doi.org/10.1111/lcrp.12135

Bennett-Levy, J. E., Butler, G. E., Fennell, M. E., Hackman, A. E., Mueller, M. E., & Westbrook, D. E. (2004). Oxford guide to behavioural experiments in cognitive therapy. Oxford University Press.

Blanchette, K., & Brown, S. L. (2006). The assessment and treatment of women offenders: An integrated perspective. John Wiley & Sons.

Blanco, C., Alegria, A. A., Petry, N. M., Grant, J., Blair Simpson, H., Liu, S.-M., Grant, B. F., & Hasin, D. (2010). Prevalence and correlates of firesetting in the US: Results from the National Epidemiologic Survey on Alcohol and Related Conditions (NESARC). *Journal of Clinical Psychiatry, 71*(9), 1218–1225. https://doi.org/10.4088/JCP.08m04812gry

Bloom, B., Owen, B., & Covington, S. (2002, November). *A theoretical basis for gender-responsive strategies in criminal justice*. In *Paper Presented at the American Society of Criminology Annual Meeting*, Chicago, IL.

Bohner, G., Reinhard, M.-A., Rutz, S., Sturm, S., Kerschbaum, B., & Effler, D. (1998). Rape myths as neutralizing cognitions: Evidence for a causal impact of anti-victim attitudes on men's self-reported likelihood of raping. *European Journal of Social Psychology, 28*(2), 257–269. https://doi.org/10.1002/(SICI)1099-0992(199803/04)28:2<257::AID-EJSP871>3.0.CO;2-1

Bonta, J., & Andrews, D. A. (2017). The psychology of criminal conduct (6th ed.). Routledge.

Bonta, J., & Wormith, J. S. (2013). Applying the risk-need-responsivity principles to offender assessment. In L. A. Craig, L. Dixon & T. A. Gannon (Eds.), What works in offender rehabilitation: An evidence-based approach to assessment and treatment (pp. 71–93). John Wiley & Sons.

Bradford, J. M. (1982). Arson: A clinical study. *Canadian Journal of Psychiatry, 27*(3), 188–193. https://doi.org/10.1177/070674378202700302

British Psychological Society (2018). *BPS code of ethics and conduct*. Retrieved from https://www.bps.org.uk/news-and-policy/bps-code-ethics-and-conduct

Brown, R., Hopkins, M., Cannings, A., & Raybould, S. (2005). Evaluation of the arson control forum's new projects initiative: Final report: January 2005: Technical annex. Office of the Deputy Prime Minister.

Brown, P., & Ross, C. (2020). Academic oversight in policy research: Questions arising from the sex offender treatment programme study. *The Lancet Psychiatry, 7*(3), 224–226. https://doi.org/10.1016/S2215-0366(19)30374-8

Brown, N., Ward, R., & Bellett, D. (2013). *An evaluation of the 'Be Firewise' programmes for year 7 and 8, and senior secondary school students (Report No. 129)*. New Zealand Fire Service Commission. https://www.fireandemergency.nz/assets/Documents/Research-and-reports/Report-129-FireWise-Evaluation-Martin-Jenkins.pdf

Budman, S. H., Soldz, S., Demby, A., Davis, M., & Merry, J. (1993). What is cohesiveness?: An empirical examination. *Small Group Research, 24*(2), 199–216. https://doi.org/10.1177/1046496493242003

Butler, H. (2018). *An investigation of scripts and dysfunctional expertise in male firesetters* [Unpublished doctoral dissertation]. University of Kent.

Butler, H., & Gannon, T. A. (2015). The scripts and expertise of firesetters: A preliminary conceptualization. *Aggression and Violent Behavior, 20*, 72–81. https://doi.org/10.1016/j.avb.2014.12.011

Butler, H., & Gannon, T. A. (2021). Do deliberate firesetters hold fire-related scripts and expertise? A quantitative investigation using fire service personnel as comparisons. *Psychology, Crime & Law, 27*(4), 383–403. https://doi.org/10.1080/1068316X.2020.1808978

Campbell, R. (2017). *Intentional fires*. National Fire Protection Association, MA. https://www.nfpa.org//-/media/Files/News-and-Research/Fire-statistics-and-reports/US-Fire-Problem/Fire-causes/osintentional.pdf

Campbell, S.-M. (2016). *A qualitative investigation of firesetting within an adult intellectually disabled population* [Unpublished doctoral dissertation]. Canterbury Christ Church University.

Canter, D., & Fritzon, K. (1998). Differentiating arsonists: A model of firesetting actions and characteristics. *Legal and Criminological Psychology, 3*(1), 73–96. https://doi.org/10.1111/j.2044-8333.1998.tb00352.x

Cassel, E., & Bernstein, D. A. (2007). Criminal Behavior (2nd ed.). Pearson.

Central Statistics Office (2016, March 30). *Recorded Crime (Quarter 4 2015)*. Retrieved September 21, 2021, from https://www.cso.ie/en/releasesandpublications/er/rc/recordedcrimequarter42015

Chanen, A., & McCutcheon, L. (2013). Prevention and early intervention for borderline personality disorder: Current status and recent evidence. *British Journal of Psychiatry, 202*(S54), S24–S29. https://doi.org/10.1192/bjp.bp.112.119180

Chen, Y. H., Arria, A. M., & Anthony, J. C. (2003). Firesetting in adolescence and being aggressive, shy, and rejected by peers: New epidemiologic evidence from a national sample survey. *Journal of the American Academy of Psychiatry and the Law Online, 31*(1), 44–52. Retrieved from http://libir.tmu.edu.tw/bitstream/987654321/17347/1/98Firesetting+in+adolescence+and+being+aggressive,+shy,+and+rejected+by+peers+new+epidemiologic+evidence+from+a+national+sample+survey.+J+Am+Acad+Psychiatry+Law.+2003%3B31(1)44-52.pdf

Chester, V., Völlm, B., Tromans, S., Kapugama, C., & Alexander, R. T. (2018). Long-stay patients with and without intellectual disability in forensic psychiatric settings: Comparison of characteristics and needs. *BJPsych Open, 4*(4), 226–234. https://doi.org/10.1192/bjo.2018.24

Clare, I. C. H., Murphy, G. M., Cox, D., & Chaplin, E. (1992). Assessment and treatment of fire-setting: A single case investigation using a cognitive-behavioural model. *Criminal Behaviour and Mental Health, 2*(3), 253–268. https://doi.org/10.1002/cbm.1992.2.3.253

Clark, L., Tyler, N., Gannon, T. A., & Kingham, M. (2014). Eye movement desensitisation and reprocessing for offence-related trauma in a mentally disordered sexual offender. *Journal of Sexual Aggression, 20*(2), 240–249. https://doi.org/10.1080/13552600.2013.822937

Clayton, P. (2000). Cognitive analytic therapy: Learning disability and firesetting. In D. Mercer, T. Mason, M. McKeown & G. McCann (Eds.), Forensic mental health care: A case study approach (pp. 12–15). Churchill Livingstone.

Coid, J. W. (1993). An affective syndrome in psychopaths with borderline personality disorder? *The British Journal of Psychiatry, 162*(5), 641–650. https://doi.org/10.1192/bjp.162.5.641

Coid, J., Kahtan, N., Gault, S., Cook, A., & Jarman, B. (2001). Medium secure forensic psychiatry services: Comparison of seven English health regions. *British Journal of Psychiatry, 178*(1), 55–61. https://doi.org/10.1192/bjp.178.1.55

Coid, J., Kahtan, N., Gault, S., & Jarman, B. (1999). Patients with personality disorder admitted to secure forensic psychiatry services. *The British Journal of Psychiatry, 175*(6), 528–536. https://doi.org/10.1192/bjp.175.6.528

Collins, J., Barnoux, M., & Langdon, P. E. (2021). Adults with intellectual disabilities and/or autism who deliberately set fires: A systematic review. *Aggression and Violent Behavior, 56*, 101545. https://doi.org/10.1016/j.avb.2020.101545

Cook, R., Hersch, R., Gaynor, J., & Roehl, J. (1989). The national juvenile firesetter/arson control and prevention programme. assessment report. The Office of Juvenile Justice and Delinquency Prevention, US Fire Administration.

Cowburn, M. (1990). Work with male sex offenders in groups. *Groupwork, 3*, 156–171.

Crime Statistics Agency Victoria (n.d.). *Spotlight: Arson Offences.* Retrieved July 8, 2021, from https://www.crimestatistics.vic.gov.au/crime-statistics/historical-crime-data/year-ending-30-september-2016/spotlight-arson-offences

Dalhuisen, L., Koenraadt, F., & Liem, M. (2017). Subtypes of firesetters. *Criminal Behaviour and Mental Health, 27*(1), 59–75. https://doi.org/10.1002/cbm.1984

Davies, J. (2019). An examination of individual versus group treatment in correctional settings. In D. L. L. Polaschek, A. Day & C. R. Hollin (Eds.), Wiley international handbook of correctional psychology (pp. 573–589). John Wiley & Sons.

De Lance, J. (1995). Gender and communication in social work education: A cross-cultural perspective. *Journal of Social Work Education, 31*(1), 75–81. https://doi.org/10.1080/1043779 7.1995.10778841

de Ruiter, C. (2018). Modifying risk factors: Building strengths. In A. R. Beech, A. J. Carter, R. E. Mann & P. Rotshtein (Eds.), The Wiley Blackwell handbook of forensic neuroscience (pp. 553–573). John Wiley & Sons.

de Vogel, V., de Ruiter, C., Bouman, Y., & de Vries Robbé, M. (2009). Guidelines for the assessment of protective factors for violence risk. Forum Educatief.

de Vries Robbé, M., & Willis, G. M. (2017). Assessment of protective factors in clinical practice. *Aggression and Violent Behavior, 32*, 55–63. https://doi.org/10.1016/j.avb.2016.12.006

Dealey, J. (2018). Moving beyond the risk paradigm: Using the good lives model with offenders in denial of sexual offending. *European Journal of Probation, 10*(1), 28–43. https://doi.org/10.1177/2066220318755530

Del Bove, G., & Mackay, S. (2011). An empirically derived classification system for juvenile firesetters. *Criminal Justice Behavior, 38*(8), 796–817. https://doi.org/10.1177/0093854811406224

Delshadian, S. (2003). Playing with fire: Art therapy in a prison setting. *Psychoanalytic Psychotherapy, 17*(1), 68–84. https://doi.org/10.1080/0266873031000096081

Dickens, G. L., Doley, R. M., & Gannon, T. A. (2016). When next? Firesetting research priorities. In R. M. Doley, G. L. Dickens & T. A. Gannon (Eds.), The psychology of arson: A practical guide to understanding and managing deliberate firesetters (pp. 290–298). Routledge.

Dickens, G. L., & Sugarman, P. (2012). Adult firesetters: Prevalence, characteristics and psychopathology. In G. L. Dickens, P. A. Sugarman & T. A. Gannon (Eds.), Firesetting and mental health (pp. 3–27). RCPsych.

Dickens, G. L., Sugarman, P., Ahmad, F., Edgar, S., Hofberg, K., & Tewari, S. (2007). Gender differences amongst adult arsonists at psychiatric assessment. *Medicine, Science and the Law, 47*(3), 233–238. https://doi.org/10.1258/rsmmsl.47.3.233

Dickens, G. L., Sugarman, P., Edgar, S., Hofberg, K., Tewari, S., & Ahmad, F. (2009). Recidivism and dangerousness in arsonists. *Journal of Forensic Psychiatry and Psychology, 20*(5), 621–639. https://doi.org/10.1080/14789940903174006

Dickens, G. L., Sugarman, P., & Gannon, T. A. (2012). Firesetting and mental health. Royal College of Psychiatrists.

Doley, R. (2009). A snapshot of serial arson in Australia. Lambert Academic Publishing (LAP).

Doley, R. M., Fineman, K., Fritzon, K., Dolan, M., & McEwan, T. E. (2011). Risk factors for recidivistic arson in adult offenders. *Psychiatry, Psychology and Law, 18*(3), 409–423. https://doi.org/10.1080/13218719.2011.559155

Douglas, J. E., Burgess, A. W., Burgess, A. G., & Ressler, R. K. (1992). Crime classification manual: A standard system for investigating and classifying violent crime. Lexington Books.

Douglas, J. E., Burgess, A. W., Burgess, A. G., & Ressler, R. K. (2006). Crime classification manual: A standard system for investigating and classifying violent crime (2nd ed.). John Wiley & Sons.

Douglas, J. E., Burgess, A. W., Burgess, A. G., & Ressler, R. K. (2013a). Crime classification manual: A standard system for investigating and classifying violent crime (3rd ed.). John Wiley & Sons.

Douglas, K. S., Hart, S. D., Webster, C. D., & Belfrage, H. (2013b). HCR-20 V3: Assessing risk for violence. Simon Fraser University.

Douglas, K. S., & Skeem, J. L. (2005). Violence risk assessment: Getting specific about being dynamic. *Psychology, Public Policy, and Law, 11*(3), 347–383. https://doi.org/10.1037/1076-8971.11.3.347

Ducat, L., McEwan, T., & Ogloff, J. R. P. (2013a). Comparing the characteristics of firesetting and non-firesetting offenders: Are firesetters a special case? *The Journal of Forensic Psychiatry & Psychology, 24*(5), 549–569. https://doi.org/10.1080/14789949.2013.821514

Ducat, L., McEwan, T., & Ogloff, J. R. P. (2015). An investigation of firesetting recidivism: Factors related to repeat offending. *Legal and Criminological Psychology, 20*(1), 1–18. https://doi.org/10.1111/lcrp.12052

Ducat, L., McEwan, T., & Ogloff, J. R. P. (2017). A comparison of psychopathology and reoffending in female and male convicted firesetters. *Law and Human Behavior, 41*(6), 588–599. https://doi.org/10.1037/lhb0000264

Ducat, L., Ogloff, J. R. P., & McEwan, T. E. (2013b). Mental illness and psychiatric treatment amongst firesetters, other offenders, and the general community. *Australian and New Zealand Journal of Psychiatry, 47*(10), 945–953. https://doi.org/10.1177/0004867413492223

Duggan, C. (2008). Focusing of treatment: The main interventions and their implications. In K. Soothill, P. Rogers & M. Dolan (Eds.), Handbook of forensic mental health (pp. 64–84). Willan Publishing.

Duggan, L., & Shine, J. (2001). An investigation of the relationship between arson, personality disorder, hostility, neuroticism and self-esteem amongst incarcerated fire-setters. *Prison Service Journal, 133*, 18–21.

Edwards, E. R. (2020). *T* [Unpublished doctoral dissertation]. University of Canterbury.

Edwards, M. J., & Grace, R. C. (2006). Analysing the offence locations and residential base of serial arsonists in New Zealand. *Australian Psychologist, 41*(3), 219–226. https://doi.org/10.1080/00050060600637626

Edwards, M. J., & Grace, R. C. (2013). The development of an actuarial model for arson recidivism. *Psychiatry, Psychology and Law, 21*(2), 218–230. https://doi.org/10.1080/13218719.2013.803277

Eisenberg, M. J., van Horn, J. E., Dekker, J. M., Assink, M., van der Put, C. E., Hendriks, J., & Stams, G. J. J. M. (2019). Static and dynamic predictors of general and violent criminal offense recidivism in the forensic outpatient population: A meta-analysis. *Criminal Justice and Behavior, 46*(5), 732–750. https://doi.org/10.1177/0093854819826109

Elbogen, E. B., & Johnson, S. C. (2009). The intricate link between violence and mental disorder: Results from the National Epidemiologic Survey on Alcohol And Related Conditions. *Archives of General Psychiatry, 66*(2), 152–161. https://doi.org/10.1001/archgenpsychiatry.2008.537

Ellison, M., Fox, C., Gains, A., & Pollock, G. (2013). An evaluation of the effect of housing provision on re-offending. *Safer Communities, 12*(1), 27–37. https://doi.org/10.1108/17578041311293125

Ellis-Smith, T., Watt, B. D., & Doley, R. M. (2019). Australian arsonists: An analysis of trends between 1990 and 2015. *Psychiatry, Psychology and Law, 26*(4), 593–613. https://doi.org/10.1080/13218719.2018.1556131

Enayati, J., Grann, M., Lubbe, S., & Fazel, S. (2008). Psychiatric morbidity in arsonists referred for forensic psychiatric assessment in Sweden. *The Journal of Forensic Psychiatry & Psychology, 19*(2), 139–147. https://doi.org/10.1080/14789940701789500

Farmer, M., McAlinden, A. M., & Maruna, S. (2016). Sex offending and situational motivation: Findings from a qualitative analysis of desistance from sexual offending. *International Journal of Offender Therapy and Comparative Criminology, 60*(15), 1756–1775. https://doi.org/10.1177/0306624X16668175

Fazel, S., & Grann, M. (2002). Older criminals: A descriptive study of psychiatrically examined offenders in Sweden. *International Journal of Geriatric Psychiatry, 17*(10), 907–913. https://doi.org/10.1002/gps.715

Federal Bureau of Investigation (2015, September 19). *Uniform crime reporting statistics: Crime in the United States, 2014.* Retrieved September 21, 2021, from https://ucr.fbi.gov/crime-in-the-u.s/2014/crime-in-the-u.s.-2014/offenses-known-to-law-enforcement/arson

Federal Bureau of Investigation. (2018a, September 10). *Uniform crime reporting statistics 2017: Crime in the United States.* Retrieved July 10, 2019, from https://ucr.fbi.gov/crime-in-the-u.s/2017/crime-in-the-u.s.-2017/tables/table-25

Federal Bureau of Investigation. (2018b, September 17). *Uniform crime report: Crime in the United States, 2017.* Retrieved September 21, 2021, from https://ucr.fbi.gov/crime-in-the-u.s/2017/crime-in-the-u.s.-2017/topic-pages/arson

Feeney, J. A., Noller, P., & Hanrahan, M. (1994). Assessing adult attachment. In M. B. Sperling & W. H. Berman (Eds.), Attachment in adults: Clinical and developmental perspectives (pp. 128–152). The Guilford Press.

Field, O. H. (2016). *Risk factors for arson recidivism in adult offenders* [Unpublished doctoral dissertation]. University of Birmingham.

Fineman, K. R. (1980). Firesetting in childhood and adolescence. *Psychiatric Clinics, 3*(3), 483–500. https://doi.org/10.1016/S0193-953X(18)30954-7

Fineman, K. R. (1995). A model for the qualitative analysis of child and adult fire deviant behavior. *American Journal of Forensic Psychology, 13*(1), 31–60. Retrieved from https://psycnet.apa.org/record/1995-29467-001

Fire and Emergency New Zealand (n.d.). *Get firewise for teachers*. Retrieved December 3, 2019, from https://www.getfirewise.org.nz

Flanagan, I. M. L., Auty, K. M., & Farrington, D. P. (2019). Parental supervision and later offending: A systematic review of longitudinal studies. *Aggression and Violent Behavior, 47*, 215–229. https://doi.org/10.1016/j.avb.2019.06.003

Fogarty, W., Lovell, M., Langenburg, J., & Heron, M.-J. (2018). *Deficit discourse and strengths-based approaches: Changing the narrative of Aboriginal and Torres Strait islander health and wellbeing*. The Lowitja Institure. https://www.lowitja.org.au/content/Document/Lowitja-Publishing/deficit-discourse-strengths-based.pdf

Freud, S. (1932). The acquisition of power over fire. *The International Journal of Psychoanalysis, 13*, 405–410. Retrieved from https://www.pep-web.org/document.php?id=IJP.013.0405A

Freud, S. (2000). *Civilisation and its discontents (electronic version, original version published in 1929)*. Chrysoma Associates Ltd. http://w3.salemstate.edu/~pglasser/Freud-Civil-Disc.pdf

Friendship, C., Falshaw, L., & Beech, A. R. (2003). Measuring the real impact of accredited offending behaviour programmes. *Legal and Criminological Psychology, 8*(1), 115–127. https://doi.org/10.1348/135532503762871282

Frisell, T., Lichtenstein, P., & Långström, N. (2011). Violent crime runs in families: A total population study of 12.5 million individuals. *Psychological Medicine, 41*(1), 97–105. https://doi.org/10.1017/S0033291710000462

Fritzon, K. (2001). An examination of the relationship between distance travelled and motivational aspects of firesetting behavior. *Journal of Environmental Psychology, 21*(1), 45–60. https://doi.org/10.1006/jevp.2000.0197

Fritzon, K., Doley, R., Davey, L., & McEwan, T. (2013). Firesetter treatment program clinician manual. Australian Centre for Arson Research and Treatment, Bond University.

Fritzon, K., Doley, R., & Hollows, K. (2014). Variations in the offence actions of deliberate firesetters: A cross national analysis. *International Journal of Offender Therapy and Comparative Criminology, 58*(10), 1150–1165. https://doi.org/10.1177/0306624X13487524

Fritzon, K., Miller, S., & Perks, D. (2022). The Psychology of fire-setting. In J. Brown & M. Horvath (Eds.), Cambridge handbook of forensic psychology (vol. *2*), 296–316. Routledge.

Gannon, T. A. (2010). Female arsonists: Key features, psychopathologies, and treatment needs. *Psychiatry: Interpersonal and Biological Processes, 73*(2), 173–189. https://doi.org/10.1521/psyc.2010.73.2.173

Gannon, T. A. (2012). *The Fire Intervention Programme for Prisoners (FIPP)* [Unpublished treatment manual for clinical provision in the Prison Service]. CORE-FP.

Gannon, T. A. (2017). *The Fire Intervention Programme for Prisoners (FIPP)* [Unpublished treatment manual for clinical provision in the Prison Service]. CORE-FP.

Gannon, T. A., Alleyne, E., Butler, H., Danby, H., Kapoor, A., Lovell, T., Mozova, K., Spruin, E., Tostevin, T., Tyler, N., & Ciardha, C. Ó. (2015). Specialist group therapy for psychological factors associated with firesetting: Evidence of a treatment effect from a non-randomized trial with male prisoners. *Behaviour Research and Therapy, 73*, 42–51. https://doi.org/10.1016/j.brat.2015.07.007

Gannon, T. A., & Barrowcliffe, E. (2012). Firesetting in the general population: The development and validation of the fire setting and fire proclivity Scales. *Legal and Criminological Psychology, 17*(1), 105–122. https://doi.org/10.1348/135532510X523203

Gannon, T. A., & Lockerbie, L. (2011). *The Firesetting Intervention Programme for Mentally Disordered Offenders (FIP-MO)* [Unpublished treatment manual for clinical provision in the NHS and Private Hospitals]. CORE-FP and Kent Forensic Psychiatry Service, NHS.

Gannon, T. A., & Lockerbie, L. (2012). *The Firesetting Intervention Programme for Mentally Disordered Offenders (FIP-MO)* [Unpublished treatment manual for clinical provision in the NHS and Private Hospitals]. CORE-FP and Kent Forensic Psychiatry Service, NHS.

Gannon, T. A., & Lockerbie, L. (2014). *The Firesetting Intervention Programme for Mentally Disordered Offenders (FIP-MO)* [Unpublished treatment manual for clinical provision in the NHS and Private Hospitals]. CORE-FP and Kent Forensic Psychiatry Service, NHS.

Gannon, T. A., & Lockerbie, L. (2017). *The Firesetting Intervention Programme for Mentally Disordered Offenders (FIP-MO)* [Unpublished treatment manual for clinical provision in the NHS and Private Hospitals]. CORE-FP and Kent Forensic Psychiatry Service, NHS.

Gannon, T. A., Ó Ciardha, C., & Barnoux, M. (2011). *The identification with fire questionnaire* [Unpublished Manuscript]. CORE-FP, School of Psychology, University of Kent.

Gannon, T. A., Ó Ciardha, C., Barnoux, M. F. L., Tyler, N., Mozova, K., & Alleyne, E. (2013). Male imprisoned firesetters have different characteristics to other imprisoned offenders and require specialist treatment. *Psychiatry: Interpersonal and Biological Processes, 76*(4), 349–364. https://doi.org/10.1521/psyc.2013.76.4.349

Gannon, T. A., Ó Ciardha, C., Doley, R. M., & Alleyne, E. (2012). The Multi-Trajectory Theory of Adult Firesetting (M-TTAF). *Aggression and Violent Behavior, 17*(2), 107–121. https://doi.org/10.1016/j.avb.2011.08.001

Gannon, T. A., Olver, M. E., Alleyne, E. K. A., Butler, H. L., Lister, V., Ó Ciardha, C., Sambrooks, K., & Tyler, N. (in preparation). *The development and validation of the Firesetting Questionnaire*. Manuscript.

Gannon, T. A., & Pina, A. (2010). Firesetting: Psychopathology, theory and treatment. *Aggression and Violent Behavior, 15*(3), 224–238. https://doi.org/10.1016/j.avb.2010.01.001

Gannon, T. A., & Ward, T. (2017). Cognition, emotion, and motivation: Future directions in sexual offending. In T. A. Gannon & T. Ward (Eds.), Sexual offending: Cognition, emotion, and motivation (pp. 127–146). Wiley-Blackwell.

Gaynor, J. (1991). Firesetting. In M. Lewis (Ed.), Child and adolescent psychiatry: A comprehensive textbook (pp. 591–603). Williams & Wilkins.

Gaynor, J., & Hatcher, C. (1987). Psychology of child firesetting. Brunner/Mazel Inc.

Geller, J. L. (1992). Communicative arson. *Hospital and Community Psychiatry, 43*(1), 76–77. https://doi.org/10.1176/ps.43.1.76

Geller, J. L., Fisher, W. H., & Moynihan, K. (1992). Adult lifetime prevalence of firesetting behaviours in a state hospital population. *Psychiatric Quarterly, 63*(2), 129–142. https://doi.org/10.1007/BF01065986

Geller, J. L., McDermeit, M., & Brown, J. M. (1997). Pyromania? What does it mean? *Journal of Forensic Science, 42*(6), 1052–1057. Retrieved from https://www.astm.org/DIGITAL_LIBRARY/JOURNALS/FORENSIC/PAGES/JFS14259J.htm

Gilbert, P. (2011). Shame in psychotherapy and the role of compassion focused therapy. In R. L. Dearing & J. P. Tangney (Eds.), Shame in the therapy hour (pp. 325–354). American Psychological Association.

Gilbert, P., & Procter, S. (2006). Compassionate mind training for people with high shame and self-criticism: Overview and pilot study of a group therapy approach. *Clinical Psychology & Psychotherapy: An International Journal of Theory & Practice, 13*(6), 353–379. https://doi.org/10.1002/cpp.507

Gobeil, R., Blanchette, K., & Stewart, L. (2016). A meta-analytic review of correctional interventions for women offenders: Gender-neutral versus gender-informed approaches. *Criminal Justice and Behavior, 43*(3), 301–322. https://doi.org/10.1177/0093854815621100

Grant, B. F., Harford, T., Dawson, D. A., Chou, P. S., & Pickering, R. P. (1995). The Alcohol Use Disorder and Associated Disabilities Interview Schedule (AUDADIS): Reliability of alcohol and drug modules in a general population sample. *Drug and Alcohol Dependence, 39*(1), 37–44. https://doi.org/10.1016/0376-8716(95)01134-K

Grant, J. E., & Kim, S. W. (2007). Clinical characteristics and psychiatric comorbidity of pyromania. *Journal of Clinical Psychiatry, 68*(11), 1717–1722. https://doi.org/10.4088/JCP.v68n1111

Green, B., Lowry, T. J., Pathé, M., & McVie, N. (2014). Firesetting patterns, symptoms and motivations of insanity acquittees charged with arson offences. *Psychiatry, Psychology and Law, 21*(6), 937–946. https://doi.org/10.1080/13218719.2014.918080

Green, B. L., Miranda, J., Daroowalla, A., & Siddique, J. (2005). Trauma exposure, mental health functioning, and program needs of women in jail. *Crime & Delinquency, 51*(1), 133–151. https://doi.org/10.1177/0011128704267477

Hagenauw, L. A., Karsten, J., Akkerman-Bouwsema, G. J., De Jager, B. E., & Lancel, M. (2015). Specific risk factors of arsonists in a forensic psychiatric hospital. *International Journal of Offender Therapy and Comparative Criminology, 59*(7), 685–700. https://doi.org/10.1177/0306624X13519744

Haines, S., Lambie, I., & Seymour, F. (2006). *International approaches to reducing deliberately lit fires: Prevention programmes* (Report No. 63). New Zealand Fire Service Commission. https://fireandemergency.nz/assets/Documents/Research-and-reports/Report-63-International-Approaches-to-Reducing-Deliberately-Lit-Fires-Prevention-Programmes.pdf

Hall, G. (1995). Using group work to understand arsonists. *Nursing Standard, 9*(23), 25–28. https://doi.org/10.7748/ns.9.23.25.s40

Hall, I., Clayton, P., & Johnson, P. (2005). Arson and learning disability. In T. Riding, C. Swann & B. Swann (Eds.), The handbook of forensic learning disability (pp. 51–52). Radcliffe Medical Press Ltd.

Hanson, R. K., & Harris, A. J. R. (2001). A structured approach to evaluating change among sexual offenders. *Sexual Abuse: A Journal of Research and Treatment, 13*, 105–122. https://doi.org/10.1023/A:1026600304489

Hanson, R. K., & Morton-Bougon, K. E. (2005). The characteristics of persistent sexual offenders: A meta-analysis of recidivism studies. *Journal of Consulting and Clinical Psychology, 73*(6), 1154–1163. https://doi.org/10.1037/0022-006X.73.6.1154

Harkins, L., & Beech, A. R. (2007). A review of the factors that can influence the effectiveness of sexual offender treatment: Risk, need, responsivity, and process issues. *Aggression and Violent Behavior, 12,* 615–627. https://doi.org/10.1016/j.avb.2006.10.006

Harkins, L., Howard, P., Barnett, G., Wakeling, H., & Miles, C. (2015). Relationships between denial, risk, and recidivism in sexual offenders. *Archives of Sexual Behavior, 44*(1), 157–166. https://doi.org/10.1007/s10508-014-0333-z

Harris, G. T., & Rice, M. E. (1996). A typology of mentally disordered firesetters. *Journal of Interpersonal Violence, 11*(3), 351–363. https://doi.org/10.1177/088626096011003003

Harris, G. T., Rice, M. E., & Quinsey, V. L. (1993). Violent recidivism of mentally disordered offenders: The development of a statistical prediction instrument. *Criminal Justice and Behavior, 20*(4), 315–335. https://doi.org/10.1177/0093854893020004001

Hart, S., Sturmey, P., Logan, C., & McMurran, M. (2011). Forensic case formulation. *International Journal of Forensic Mental Health, 10*(2), 118–126. https://doi.org/10.1080/149 99013.2011.577137

Heffernan, R., & Ward, T. (2017). A comprehensive theory of dynamic risk and protective factors. *Aggression and Violent Behavior, 37,* 129–141. https://doi.org/10.1016/j. avb.2017.10.003

Henretty, J. R., Currier, J. M., Berman, J. S., & Levitt, H. M. (2014). The impact of counselor self-disclosure on clients: A meta-analytic review of experimental and quasi-experimental research. *Journal of Counseling Psychology, 61*(2), 191–207. https://doi.org/10.1037/a0036189

Henretty, J. R., & Levitt, H. M. (2010). The role of therapist self-disclosure in psychotherapy: A qualitative review. *Clinical Psychology Review, 30*(1), 63–77. https://doi.org/10.1016/j. cpr.2009.09.004

Hill, C. E., Knox, S., & Pinto-Coelho, K. G. (2018). Therapist self-disclosure and immediacy: A qualitative meta-analysis. *Psychotherapy, 55*(4), 445–460. https://doi.org/10.1037/pst0000182

Hoertel, N., Le Strat, Y., Schuster, J.-P., & Limosin, F. (2011). Gender difference in firesetting: Results from the National Epidemiologic Survey on Alcohol and Related Conditions (NESARC). *Psychiatry Research, 190*(2-3), 352–358. https://doi.org/10.1016/j. psychres.2011.05.045

Holbrook, T. L., Hoyt, D. B., Stein, M. B., & Sieber, W. J. (2002). Gender differences in long-term posttraumatic stress disorder outcomes after major trauma: Women are at higher risk of adverse outcomes than men. *Journal of Trauma and Acute Care Surgery, 53*(5), 882–888. https://doi.org/10.1097/01.TA.0000033749.65011.6A

Hollin, C. R., Davies, S., Duggan, C., Huband, N., McCarthy, L., & Clarke, M. (2013). Patients with a history of arson admitted to medium security: Characteristics on admission and follow-up post-discharge. *Medicine, Science and the Law, 53*(3), 154–160. https://doi. org/10.1258/msl.2012.012056

Home Office (2021, September 16). *Fire statistics data tables: Deliberate fires attended.* Retrieved September 21, 2021, from https://www.gov.uk/government/statistical-data-sets/ fire-statistics-data-tables#deliberate-fires-attended

Hooker, C. A. (1987). A realistic theory of science. State University of NY.

Horsley, F. (2020). *Arson reconceptualised: The continuum of fire use* [Unpublished doctoral dissertation]. University of Durham.

Hosmer, D. W., Jr., Lemeshow, S., & Sturdivant, R. X. (2013). Applied Logistic Regression (3rd ed.). John Wiley & Sons, Inc.

Howard, M. V. A., de Almeida Neto, A. C., & Galouzis, J. J. (2018). Relationships between treatment delivery, program attrition, and reoffending outcomes in an intensive custodial sex offender program. *Sexual Abuse, 31*(4), 477–499. https://doi.org/10.1177/1079063218764886

Howlett, L., Flint, K., Deal, K., Dudley, A., Horn, T., Langan, G., Jeczalik, J. J., & Morley, P. (1997). Firestarter [Recorded by The Prodigy]. On The fat of the land [CD]. XL Recordings.

Hwang, V., Duchossois, G. P., Garcia-Espana, J. F., & Durbin, D. R. (2006). Impact of a community based fire prevention intervention on fire safety knowledge and behaviour in elementary school children. *Injury Prevention, 12*(5), 344–346. https://doi.org/10.1136/ip.2005.011197

Icove, D. J., & Estepp, M. H. (1987). Motive-based offender profiles of arson and fire-related crimes. *FBI Law Enforcement Bulletin, 56*, 17–23. Retrieved from https://heinonline.org/HOL/Page?handle=hein.journals/fbileb56&div=35&id=&page=&collection=journals

Imhoff, R. (2015). Punitive attitudes against pedophiles or persons with sexual interest in children: Does the label matter? *Archives of Sexual Behavior, 44*(1), 35–44. https://doi.org/10.1007/s10508-014-0439-3

Inciardi, J. A. (1970). The adult firesetter: A typology. *Criminology, 8*(2), 145–155. https://doi.org/10.1111/j.1745-9125.1970.tb00736.x

Ingamells, B., & Morrissey, C. (2014). I Can Feel Good: Skills training for people with intellectual disabilities and problems managing emotions. Pavilion Publishing and Media Ltd.

Jackson, H. F. (1994). Assessment of fire-setters. In M. McMurran & J. Hodge (Eds.), The assessment of criminal behaviours in secure settings (pp. 94–126). Jessica Kingsley.

Jackson, H. F., Glass, C., & Hope, S. (1987). A functional analysis of recidivistic arson. *British Journal of Clinical Psychology, 26*(3), 175–185. https://doi.org/10.1111/j.2044-8260.1987.tb01345.x

Kalmar, D., & Sternberg, R. (1988). Theory knitting: An integrative approach to theory development. *Philosophical Psychology, 1*(2), 153–170. https://doi.org/10.1080/09515088808572934

Karterud, S. W., & Kongerslev, M. T. (2019). A Temperament-Attachment-Mentalization-Based (TAM) theory of personality and its disorders. *Frontiers in Psychology, 10*, 518. https://doi.org/10.3389/fpsyg.2019.00518

Kaufman, I., Heims, L. W., & Reiser, D. E. (1961). A reevaluation of the psychodynamics of firesetting. *American Journal of Orthopsychiatry, 31*(1), 123–136. https://doi.org/10.1111/j.1939-0025.1961.tb02113.x

Ketola, J., & Kokki, E. (2018). *Finnish Rescue Services' Pocket Statistics 2013-2017*. http://info.smedu.fi/kirjasto/Sarja_D/D3_2018.pdf

Kim, D.-Y., Joo, H.-J., & McCarty, W. P. (2008). Risk assessment and classification of day reporting center clients: An actuarial approach. *Criminal Justice and Behavior, 35*(6), 792–812. https://doi.org/10.1177/0093854808315067

Kocsis, R. N., & Cooksey, R. W. (2002). Criminal psychological profiling of serial arson crimes. *International Journal of Offender Therapy and Comparative Criminology, 46*(6), 631–656. https://doi.org/10.1177/0306624X02238159

Kolko, D. J. (2002). Handbook on firesetting in children and youth. Elsevier.

Kolko, D. J., & Kazdin, A. E. (1992). The emergence and recurrence of child firesetting: A one-year prospective study. *Journal of Abnormal Child Psychology, 20*(1), 17–37. https://doi.org/10.1007/bf00927114

Kolko, D. J., Scharf, D. M., Herschell, A. D., Wilcox, D. K., Okulitch, J., & Pinsonneault, I. (2008). A survey of juvenile firesetter intervention programs in North America. *American Journal of Forensic Psychology, 26*(4), 41–66.

Koson, D. F., & Dvoskin, J. (1982). Arson: A diagnostic study. *Bulletin of the American Academy of Psychiatry and Law, 10*(1), 39–49. Retrieved from http://jaapl.org/content/jaapl/10/1/39.full.pdf

Kroner, D. G., & Mills, J. F. (2002). *The criminal attribution inventory: User guide.* Unpublished instrument and user guide.

Kroner, D. G., & Yessine, A. K. (2013). Changing risk factors that impact recidivism: In search of mechanisms of change. *Law and Human Behavior, 37*(5), 321–336. https://doi.org/10.1037/lhb00000022

Lambie, I., Best, C., Tran, H., Ioane, J., & Shepherd, M. (2015). Risk factors for fire injury in school leavers: A review of the literature. *Fire Safety Journal, 77*, 59–66. https://doi.org/10.1016/j.firesaf.2015.07.004

Lambie, I., Best, C., Tran, H., Ioane, J., & Shepherd, M. (2018). Evaluating effective methods of engaging school leavers in adopting safety behavours. *Fire Safety Journal, 96*, 134–142. https://doi.org/10.1016/j.firesaf.2017.11.011

Lande, S. D. (1980). A combination of orgasmic reconditioning and overt sensitisation in the treatment of a fire fetish. *Journal of Behavioural Therapy and Experimental Psychiatry, 11*(4), 291–296. https://doi.org/10.1016/0005-7916(80)90075-0

Lehna, C., Coty, M. B., Fahey, E., Williams, J., Scrivener, D., Wishnia, G., & Myers, J. (2015b). Intervention study for changes in home fire safety knowledge in urban older adults. *Burns, 41*(6), 1205–1211. https://doi.org/10.1016/j.burns.2015.02.012

Lehna, C., Fahey, E., Janes, E. G., Rengers, S., Williams, J., Scrivener, D., & Myers, J. (2015a). Home fire safety education for parents of newborns. *Burns, 41*(6), 1199–1204. https://doi.org/10.1016/j.burns.2015.02.009

Lehna, C., Merrell, J., Furmanek, S., & Twyman, S. (2017). Home fire safety intervention pilot with urban older adults living in Wales. *Burns, 43*(1), 69–75. https://doi.org/10.1016/j.burns.2016.06.025

Levenson, J. (2014). Incorporating trauma-informed care into evidence-based sex offender treatment. *Journal of Sexual Aggression, 20*(1), 9–22. https://doi.org/10.1080/13552600.2013.861523

Levin, B. (1976). Psychological characteristics of firesetters. *Fire Journal, 70*(2), 36–41. Retrieved from https://psycnet.apa.org/record/1977-12965-001

Lewis, N. D. C., & Yarnell, H. (1951). Pathological firesetting; Pyromania. Nervous and Mental Disease Monographs.

Lindberg, N., Holi, M. M., Tani, P., & Virkkunen, M. (2005). Looking for pyromania: Characteristics of a consecutive sample of Finnish male criminals with histories of recidivist fire-setting between 1973 and 1993. *BMC Psychiatry, 5*(47), 1–5. https://doi.org/10.1186/1471-244X-5-47

Linehan, M. M. (2015). DBT? Skills Training Manual (2nd ed.). The Guildford Press.

Lipsey, M., Ladenberger, N. A., & Wilson, S. J. (2007). Effects of cognitive behavioural programs for criminal offenders. *Campbell Systematic Reviews, 3*(1), 1–27. https://doi.org/10.4073/csr.2007.6

Logan, C. (2014). The HCR-20 version 3: A case study in risk formulation. *International Journal of Forensic Mental Health, 13*(2), 1–9. https://doi.org/10.1080/14999013.2014.906516

Logan, C., Brown, P., & Martin, J. (2010, January). *Firesetting risk assessment and management: A structured professional judgement approach.* In *Paper presented at Rampton Hospital,* Woodbeck, Nottinghamshire, UK.

Long, C. G., Banyard, E., Fulton, B., & Hollin, C. R. (2013). Developing an assessment of fire-setting to guide treatment in secure settings: The St Andrew's Fire and Arson Risk Instrument (SAFARI). *Behavioural and Cognitive Psychotherapy, 42,* 617–628. https://doi.org/10.1017/S1352465813000477

Long, C. G., Dickens, G., & Dolley, O. (2014). Features and motivators of emotionally expressive firesetters: The assessment of women in secure psychiatric settings. *Journal of Criminal Psychology, 4*(2), 129–142. https://doi.org/10.1108/JCP-08-2013-0022

Long, C. G., Fitzgerald, K.-A., & Hollin, C. R. (2015). Women firesetters admitted to secure psychiatric services: Characteristics and treatment needs. *Victims & Offenders, 10*(3), 341–353. https://doi.org/10.1080/15564886.2014.967901

MacDonald, J. M. (1963). The threat to kill. *American Journal of Psychiatry, 120*(2), 125–130. https://doi.org/10.1176/ajp.120.2.125

Macht, L. B., & Mack, J. E. (1968). The firesetter syndrome. *Psychiatry, 31*(3), 277–288. https://doi.org/10.1080/00332747.1968.11023556

Mann, R. E., Webster, S. D., Schofield, C., & Marshall, W. L. (2004). Approach versus avoidance goals in relapse prevention with sexual offenders. *Sexual Abuse: A Journal of Research and Treatment, 16,* 65–75. https://doi.org/10.1023/B:SEBU.0000006285.73534.57

Marshall, W. L., & Burton, D. L. (2010). The importance of group processes in offender treatment. *Aggression and Violent Behavior, 15*(2), 141–149. https://doi.org/10.1016/j.avb.2009.08.008

Marshall, W. L., Marshall, L. E., & Burton, D. L. (2013). Feautrues of treatment delivery and group processes that maximize the effects of offender programs. In J. L. Wood & T. A. Gannon (Eds.), Crime and crime reduction: The importance of group processes (pp. 159–176). Routledge.

Marshall, W. L., Marshall, L. E., Serran, G. A., & O'Brien, M. D. (2011). Rehabilitating sexual offenders: A strength-based approach. American Psychological Association.

Marshall, W. L., Serran, G. A., Fernandez, Y. M., Mulloy, R., Mann, R. E., & Thornton, D. (2003). Therapist characteristics in the treatment of sexual offenders: Tentative data on their relationship with indices of behavior change. *Journal of Sexual Aggression, 9,* 25–30. https://doi.org/10.1080/355260031000137940

Marshall, W. L., Serran, G., Marshall, L. E., & Fernandez, Y. M. (2005). Recovering memories of the offense in" amnesic" sexual offenders. *Sexual Abuse, 17*(1), 31–38. https://doi.org/10.1177/107906320501700104

Marshall, W. L., Serran, G. A., Moulden, H., Mulloy, R., Fernandez, Y. M., Mann, R. E., & Thornton, D. (2002). Therapist features in sexual offender treatment: Their reliable identification and influence on behavior change. *Clinical Psychology and Psychotherapy, 9*(6), 395–405. https://doi.org/10.1002/cpp.335

Marshall, W. L., Thornton, D., Marshall, L. E., Fernandez, Y. M., & Mann, R. (2001). Treatment of sexual offenders who are in categorical denial: A pilot project. *Sexual Abuse: A Journal of Research and Treatment, 13*, 205–215. https://doi.org/10.1023/A:1009540301151

Maruna, S., & Mann, R. E. (2006). A fundamental attribution error? Rethinking cognitive distortions. *Legal and Criminological Psychology, 11*(2), 155–177. https://doi.org/10.1348/135532506X114608

Mayhew, P. (2003). *Counting the costs of crime in Australia (Trends & Issues in Crime and Criminal Justice No. 247)*. Australian Institute of Criminology. https://aic.gov.au/publications/tandi/tandi247

Mayo Clinic (2016, September 23). *Personality disorders*. Retrieved January 18, 2020, from https://www.mayoclinic.org/diseases-conditions/personality-disorders/symptoms-causes/syc-20354463

McCarty, C. A., & McMahon, R. J. (2005). Domains of risk in the developmental continuity of fire setting. *Behavior Therapy, 36*(2), 185–195. https://doi.org/10.1016/S0005-7894(05)80067-X

McEwan, T. E., & Ducat, L. (2016). The role of mental disorder in firesetting behaviour. In R. M. Doley, G. L. Dickens & T. A. Gannon (Eds.), The psychology of arson: A practical guide to understanding and managing deliberate firesetters (pp. 211–227). Routledge.

McMurran, M., & Theodosi, E. (2007). Is treatment non-completion associated with increased reconviction over no treatment? *Psychology, Crime & Law, 13*(4), 333–343. https://doi.org/10.1080/10683160601060374

Meacham, B. J. (2020). *Developing a global standard for fire reporting*. Retrieved from Royal Institution of Chartered Surveyors, London, UK https://www.rics.org/globalassets/rics-website/media/knowledge/research/insights/developing-a-global-standard-for-fire-reporting.pdf

Mews, A., Di Bella, L., & Purver, M. (2017). Impact evaluation of the prison-based core sex offender treatment programme. Ministry of Justice.

Miller, J. B. (1976). Toward a new psychology of women. Beacon Press.

Miller, S., & Fritzon, K. (2007). Functional consistency across two behavioural modalities: Fire-setting and self-harm in female special hospital patients. *Criminal Behaviour and Mental Health, 17*(1), 31–44. https://doi.org/10.1002/cbm.637

Mills, J. F., & Kroner, D. G. (2001). *Measures of Criminal Attitudes and Associates (MCAA)* [Unpublished instrument and user guide]. https://doi.org/10.13140/2.1.4785.4081

Muckley, A. (1997). Firesetting: Addressing offending behaviour. A resource and training manual. Redcar and Cleveland Psychological Service.

Muller, D., & Stebbins, A. (2007). Juvenile arson intervention programs in Australia. *Trends & Issues in Crime and Criminal Justice, 335*, 1–6. Retrieved from https://www.aic.gov.au/publications/bfab/bfab3

Murphy, G. H., & Clare, I. C. (1996). Analysis of motivation in people with mild learning disabilities (mental handicap) who set fires. *Psychology, Crime and Law, 2*(3), 153–164. https://doi.org/10.1080/10683169608409774

Nanayakkara, V., Ogloff, J. R. P., Davis, M. R., & McEwan, T. E. (2020a). Gender-based types of firesetting: Clinical, behavioural and motivational differences among female and male firesetters. *The Journal of Forensic Psychiatry & Psychology, 31*(2), 273–291. https://doi.org/10.1080/14789949.2020.1720266

Nanayakkara, V., Ogloff, J. R. P., McEwan, T. E., & Davis, M. R. (2020b). Applying classification methodology to high-consequence firesetting. *Psychology, Crime & Law, 26*(7), 1–23. https://doi.org/10.1080/1068316X.2020.1733568

Nanayakkara, V., Ogloff, J. R. P., McEwan, T. E., & Ducat, L. (2020c). Firesetting among people with mental disorders: Differences in diagnosis, motives and behaviour. *International Journal of Forensic Mental Health*. Advanced online publication. https://doi.org/10.1080/14999013.2020.1830891

Nanayakkara, V., Ogloff, J. R. P., & Thomas, S. D. M. (2015). From haystacks to hospitals: An evolving understanding of mental disorder and firesetting. *International Journal of Forensic Mental Health, 14*(1), 66–75. https://doi.org/10.1080/14999013.2014.974086

National Institute for Health and Care Excellence (NICE) (2018, December 5). *Post-traumatic stress disorder*. Retrieved March 4, 2021, from https://www.nice.org.uk/guidance/ng116

Noblett, S., & Nelson, B. (2001). A psychosocial approach to arson – A case controlled study of female offenders. *Medicine, Science and the Law, 41*(4), 325–330. https://doi.org/10.1177/002580240104100409

Novaco, R. W. (2003). The Novaco anger scale and provocation inventory: NAS-PI. Western Psychological Services.

Nowicki, S., Jr. (1976). Adult Nowicki-Strickland internal-external locus of control scale. Test Manual available from S. Nowicki, Jr., Department of Psychology, Emory University, 30322.

Ó Ciardha, C. (2015). The relationship between firesetting and sexual offending. In R. Doley, G. L. Dickens & T. A. Gannon (Eds.), The psychology of arson: A practical guide to understanding and managing deliberate firesetters (pp. 198–207). Routledge.

Ó Ciardha, C. (2016). The relationship between firesetting and sexual offending. In R. M. Doley, G. L. Dickens & T. A. Gannon (Eds.), The psychology of arson: A practical guide to understanding and managing deliberate firesetters (pp. 198–207). Routledge.

Ó Ciardha, C., Alleyne, E. K., Tyler, N., Barnoux, M. F., Mozova, K., & Gannon, T. A. (2015a). Examining the psychopathology of incarcerated male firesetters using the millon clinical multiaxial inventory-III. *Psychology, Crime & Law, 21*(6), 606–616. https://doi.org/10.1080/1068316X.2015.1008478

Ó Ciardha, C., Barnoux, M. F. L., Alleyne, E. K. A., Tyler, N., Mozova, K., & Gannon, T. A. (2015b). Multiple factors in the assessment of firesetters' fire interest and attitudes. *Legal and Criminological Psychology, 20*(1), 37–47. https://doi.org/10.111/lcrp.12065

Ó Ciardha, C., & Gannon, T. A. (2012). The implicit theories of firesetters: A preliminary conceptualization. *Aggression and Violent Behavior, 17*(2), 122–128. https://doi.org/10.1016/j.avb.2011.12.001

Ó Ciardha, C., Tyler, N., & Gannon, T. A. (2015c). A practical guide to assessing adult firesetters' fire-specific treatment needs using the four factor fire scales. *Psychiatry: Interpersonal and Biological Processes, 78*(4), 293–304. https://doi.org/10.1080/00332747.2015.1061310

Ó Ciardha, C., Tyler, N., & Gannon, T. A. (2017). Pyromania. In S. Goldstein & M. DeVries (Eds.), Handbook of DSM-5 disorders in children and adolescents (pp. 529–538). Springer International Publishing.

O'Meara, A., Edwards, M., & Davies, J. (2020). Listening to women: Relational approaches to female offender management. *The Journal of Forensic Practice, 23*(1), 1–12. https://doi.org/10.1108/JFP-06-2020-0025

Ogier, S. (2008). *Evaluation of the firewise programme for year one and two students (Report No. 81)*. New Zealand Fire Service Commission. https://www.fireandemergency.nz/assets/Documents/Research-and-reports/Report-81-Evaluation-of-Firewise-Programmes.pdf

Olver, M. E., Stockdale, K. C., & Wormith, J. S. (2011). A meta-analysis of predictors of offender treatment attrition and its relationship to recidivism. *Journal of Consulting and Clinical Psychology, 79*(1), 6–21. https://doi.org/10.1037/a0022200

Palmer, E., Caulfield, L. S., & Hollin, C. R. (2005). Evaluation of interventions with arsonists and young firesetters. Office of the Deputy Prime Minister.

Parfitt, C. H., & Alleyne, E. (2020). Not the sum of its parts: A critical review of the MacDonald Triad. *Trauma, Violence, and Abuse, 21*(2), 300–310. https://doi.org/10.1177/1524838018764164

Parks, R. W., Green, R. D. J., Girgis, S., Hunter, M. D., Woodruff, P. W. R., & Spence, S. A. (2005). Response of pyromania to biological treatment in a homeless person. *Neuropsychiatric Disease and Treatment, 1*(3), 277–280. Retrieved from https://www.ncbi.nlm.nih.gov/pmc/articles/PMC2416759/pdf/ndt-0103-277.pdf

Patton, J. H., Stanford, M. S., & Barratt, E. S. (1995). Factor structure of the Barratt impulsiveness scale. *Journal of Clinical Psychology, 51*(6), 768–774. https://doi.org/10.1002/1097-4679(199511)51:6768::AID-JCLP22705106073.0.CO;2-1

Peluso, P. R., & Freund, R. R. (2018). Therapist and client emotional expression and psychotherapy outcomes: A meta-analysis. *Psychotherapy, 55*(4), 461–472. https://doi.org/10.1037/pst0000165

Perks, D. L. C., Watt, B. D., Fritzon, K., & Doley, R. M. (2019). Juvenile firesetters as multiple problem youth with particular interests in fire: A meta-analysis. *Aggression and Violent Behavior, 47*, 189–203. https://doi.org/10.1016/j.avb.2019.04.003

Piper, W. E., Marrache, M., Lacroix, R., Richardsen, A. M., & Jones, B. D. (1983). Cohesion as a basic bond in groups. *Human Relations, 36*(2), 93–108. https://doi.org/10.1177/001872678303600201

Pollock, P. (2006). From theory to practice: Cognitive analytic therapy for an arsonist with borderline personality disorder. In P. H. Pollock, M. Stowell-Smith & M. Göpfert (Eds.), Cognitive analytic therapy for offenders: A new approach to forensic psychotherapy (pp. pp. 43–65). Routledge.

Porter, C., Palmier-Claus, J., Branitsky, A., Mansell, W., Warwick, H., & Varese, F. (2020). Childhood adversity and borderline personality disorder: A meta-analysis. *Acta Psychiatrica Scandinavica, 141*(1), 6–20. https://doi.org/10.1111/acps.13118

Prins, H. (1994). Fire-raising: Its motivation and management. Routledge.

Quinsey, V. L., Chaplin, T. C., & Upfold, D. (1989). Arsonists and sexual arousal to fire setting: Correlation unsupported. *Journal of Behavior Therapy and Experimental Psychiatry, 20*(3), 203–209. https://doi.org/10.1016/0005-7916(89)90024-4

Räsänen, P., Hakko, H., & Väisänen, E. (1995). The mental state of arsonists as determined by forensic psychiatric examinations. *Journal of the American Academy of Psychiatry and the Law Online, 23*(4), 547–553. Retrieved from https://www.researchgate.net/profile/Helinae-Hakko/publication/14560545_The_mental_states_of_arsonists_as_determined_by_psychiatric_ examinations/links/09e415136f7bd469e3000000/The-mental-states-of-arsonists-as-determined-by-psychiatric-examinations.pdf

Räsänen, P., Puumalainen, T., Janhonen, S., & Väisänen, E. (1996). Fire-setting from the viewpoint of an arsonist. *Journal of Psychosocial Nursing and Mental Health Services, 34*(3), 16–21. https://doi.org/10.3928/0279-3695-19960301-14

Raynor, P. (2007). Risk and need assessment in British probation: The contribution of the LSI-R. *Psychology, Crime and Law, 13*(2), 125–138. https://doi.org/10.1080/10683160500337592

Rees-Jones, A. (2011). *Examining the utility of assessment tools and group intervention programmes for mentally disordered offenders* [Unpublished doctoral dissertation]. The Centre for Forensic and Criminological Psychology, University of Birmingham.

Reichborn-Kjennerud, T., Czajkowski, N., Ystrøm, E., Ørstavik, R., Aggen, S. H., Tambs, K., Torgersen, S., Neale, M. C., Røysamb, E., Krueger, R. F., Knudsen, G. P., & Kendler, K. S. (2015). A longitudinal twin study of borderline and antisocial personality disorder traits in early to middle adulthood. *Psychological Medicine, 45*(14), 3121–3131. https://doi.org/10.1017/S0033291715001117

Repo, E., Virkkunen, M., Rawlings, R., & Linnoila, M. (1997). Criminal and psychiatric histories of Finnish arsonists. *Acta Psychiatrica Scandinavia, 95*(4), 318–323. https://doi.org/10.1111/j.1600-0447.1997.tb09638.x

Rice, M. E., & Chaplin, T. C. (1979). Social skills training for hospitalized male arsonists. *Journal of Behavior Therapy and Experimental Psychiatry, 10*(2), 105–108. https://doi.org/10.1016/0005-7916(79)90083-1

Rice, M. E., & Harris, G. T. (1991). Firesetters admitted to a maximum security psychiatric institution: Offenders and offenses. *Journal of Interpersonal Violence, 6*(4), 461–475. https://doi.org/10.1177/088626091006004005

Rice, M. E., & Harris, G. T. (1996). Predicting the recidivism of mentally disordered firesetters. *Journal of Interpersonal Violence, 11*(3), 364–375. https://doi.org/10.1177/088626096011003004

Rice, M. E., & Harris, G. T. (2008). Arson. In V. N. Parrillo (Ed.), The encyclopedia of social problems (pp. 56–57). Sage Publications Inc.

Rimé, B. (2007). The social sharing of emotion as an interface between individual and collective processes in the construction of emotional climates. *Journal of Social Issues, 63*(2), 307–322. https://doi.org/10.1111/j.1540-4560.2007.00510.x

Rimé, B. (2009). Emotion elicits the social sharing of emotion: Theory and empirical review. *Emotion Review, 1*(1), 60–85. https://doi.org/10.1177/1754073908097189

Ritchie, E. C., & Huff, T. G. (1999). Psychiatric aspects of arsonists. *Journal of Forensic Science, 44*(4), 733–740. https://doi.org/10.1520/jfs14546j

Rix, K. J. B. (1994). A psychiatric study of adult arsonists. *Medicine Science and the Law, 34*(1), 21–34. https://doi.org/10.1177/002580249403400104

Root, C., MacKay, S., Henderson, J., Del Bove, G., & Warling, D. (2008). The link between maltreatment and juvenile firesetting: Correlates and underlying mechanisms. *Child Abuse and Neglect, 32*(2), 161–176. https://doi.org/10.1016/j.chiabu.2007.07.004

Ross, T., & Pfäfflin, F. (2007). Attachment and interpersonal problems in a prison environment. *Journal of Forensic Psychiatry and Psychology, 18*(1), 90–98. https://doi.org/10.1080/14789940601063345

Roy, A., Virkkunen, M., Guthrie, S., & Linnoila, M. (1986). Indices of serotonin and glucose metabolism in violent offenders, arsonists and alcoholics. In J. J. Mann & M. Stanley (Eds.), Psychology of suicidal behavior (pp. 202–220). Academy of Sciences.

Royer, F. L., Flynn, W. F., & Osadca, B. H. (1971). Case history: Aversion therapy for fire setting by a deteriorated schizophrenic. *Behavior Therapy, 2*(2), 229–232. https://doi.org/10.1016/S0005-7894(71)80010-2

Ruocco, A. C., & Carcone, D. (2016). A neurobiological model of borderline personality disorder: Systematic and integrative review. *Harvard Review of Psychiatry, 24*(5), 311–329. https://doi.org/10.1097/HRP.0000000000000123

Salo, B., Laaksonen, T., & Santtila, P. (2019). Predictive power of dynamic (vs. static) risk factors in the Finnish risk and needs assessment form. *Criminal Justice and Behavior, 46*(7), 939–960. https://doi.org/10.1177/0093854819848793

Sambrooks, K. (2021). *Virtual reality firesetting assessment* [Unpublished raw data].

Sambrooks, K., Olver, M. E., Page, T. E., & Gannon, T. A. (2021). Firesetting reoffending: A meta-analysis. *Criminal Justice and Behavior*. Advanced online publication. https://doi.org/10.1177/00938548211013577

Sambrooks, K., & Tyler, N. (2019). What works with adult deliberate firesetters? Where have we come from and where do we go from here? *Forensic Update, 130*, 17–20. Retrieved from https://research.kent.ac.uk/fire-intervention-programme/wp-content/uploads/sites/1356/2019/07/what-works-with-adult-deliberate-firesetters.pdf

Sapsford, R. J., Banks, C., & Smith, D. D. (1978). Arsonists in prison. *Medicine, Science, and Law, 18*(4), 247–264. https://doi.org/10.1177/002580247801800405

Schindler, S. (2018). Theoretical virtues in science: Uncovering reality through science. Cambridge University Press.

Scott, D. (1974). The psychology of fire. Charles Scribner's Sons.

Seidler, G. H., & Wagner, F. E. (2006). Comparing the efficacy of EMDR and trauma- focussed cognitive behavioral therapy in the treatment of PTSD: A meta-analytic study. *Psychological Medicine, 36*(11), 1515–1522. https://doi.org/10.1017/S0033291706007963

Sentencing Council (2018, March 27). *Statistical bulletin: Arson and criminal damage offences.* Retrieved January 20, 2020, from https://www.sentencingcouncil.org.uk/wp-content/uploads/Arson-and-criminal-damage-statistical-bulletin-1.pdf

Serin, R. C., Chadwick, N., & Lloyd, C. D. (2016). Dynamic risk and protective factors. *Psychology, Crime and Law, 22*(1-2), 151–170. https://doi.org/10.1080/1068316X.2016.1112013

Serran, G. (2017). Cognition, emotion and motivation: Treatment for individuals who have sexually offended. In T. A. Gannon & T. Ward (Eds.), Sexual offending: Cognition, emotion, and motivation (pp. 109–126). Wiley-Blackwell.

Serran, G., Fernandez, Y., Marshall, W. L., & Mann, R. E. (2003). Process issues in treatment: Application to sexual offender programs. *Professional Psychology: Research and Practice, 34*(4), 368–374. https://doi.org/10.1037/0735-7028.34.4.368

Simmons, J. P., Nelson, L. D., & Simonsohn, U. (2021). Pre-registration: Why and how. *Journal of Consumer Psychology, 31*(1), 151–162. https://doi.org/10.1002/jcpy.1208

Singh, J. P., Desmarais, S. L., Hurducas, C., Arbach-Lucioni, K., Condemarin, C., Dean, K., Doyle, M., Folino, J. O., Godoy-Cervera, V., Grann, M., Ho, R. M. Y., Large, M. M., Hjort Nielsen, L., Pham, T. H., Rebocho, M. F., Reeves, K. A., Rettenberger, M., de Ruiter, C., Seewald, K., & Otto, R. K. (2014). International perspectives on the practical application of violence risk assessment: A global survey of 44 countries. *International Journal of Forensic Mental Health, 13*(3), 193–206. https://doi.org/10.1080/14999013.2014.922141

Skoglund, C., Tiger, A., Rück, C., Petrovic, P., Asherson, P., Hellner, C., Mataix-Cols, M., & Kuja-Halkola, R. (2019). Familial risk and heritability of diagnosed borderline personality disorder: A register study of the Swedish population. *Molecular Psychiatry, 26*(3), 1–10. https://doi.org/10.1038/s41380-019-0442-0

Slavkin, M. L. (2000). *Juvenile firesetters: An exploratory analysis* [Unpublished doctoral dissertation]. Indiana University.

Smith, R. G., Jorna, P., Sweeney, J., & Fuller, G. (2014). *Counting the costs of crime in Australia: A 2011 estimate* (Research and Public Policy Series No. 129). Australian Institute of Criminology. https://www.aic.gov.au/publications/rpp/rpp129

Smith, J., & Short, J. (1995). Mentally disordered firesetters. *British Journal of Hospital Medicine, 53*(4), 136–140. https://pubmed.ncbi.nlm.nih.gov/7735661

Soothill, K., Ackerly, E., & Francis, B. (2004). The criminal careers of arsonists. *Medicine, Science and the Law, 44*(1), 27–40. https://doi.org/10.1258/rsmmsl.44.1.27

Soothill, K. L., & Pope, P. J. (1973). Arson: A twenty-year cohort study. *Medicine, Science, and the Law, 13*(2), 127–138. https://doi.org/10.1177/002580247301300211

Statistics Canada (2019, July 22). *Incident-based crime statistics, by detailed violations, Canada, provinces, territories, and Cencus Metropoliton areas.* Retrieved November 11, 2019, from https://www150.statcan.gc.ca/t1/tbl1/en/tv.action?pid=3510017701&pickMembers%5B0%5D=1.1&pickMembers%5B1%5D=2.84

Statistics Canada (2021, July 27). *Incident-based crime statistics, by detailed violations, Canada, provinces, territories, and Cencus Metropoliton areas.* Retrieved July 8, 2021, from https://www150.statcan.gc.ca/t1/tbl1/en/tv.action?pid=3510017701

Stewart, L. A. (1993). Profile of female firesetters. Implications for treatment. *British Journal of Psychiatry, 163*(2), 248–256. https://doi.org/10.1192/bjp.163.2.248

Strauss, A. L., & Corbin, J. M. (1998). Basics of qualitative research and techniques and procedures for developing grounded theory (2nd ed.). Sage Publications.

Strub, D. S., Douglas, K. S., & Nicholls, T. L. (2014). The validity of the version 3 of the HCR-20 violence risk assessment scheme amongst offenders and civil psychiatric patients. *International Journal of Forensic Mental Health, 13*(2), 148–159. https://doi.org/10.1080/14999013.2014.911785

Sturmey, P., & McMurran, M. (2011). Forensic case formulation. John Wiley & Sons, Ltd.

Swaffer, T., Haggett, M., & Oxley, T. (2001). Mentally disordered firesetters: A structured intervention programme. *Clinical Psychology and Psychotherapy, 8*(6), 468–475. https://doi.org/10.1002/cpp.299

Taylor, J. L. (2014, October). *Roots, referrals, risks and remedies for offenders with intellectual disabilities. Paper Presented at A Risky Business, BPS Conference,* University of Manchester, Manchester, UK.

Taylor, J. L., Robertson, A., Thorne, I., Belshaw, T., & Watson, A. (2006). Responses of female fire-setters with mild and borderline intellectual disabilities to a group intervention. *Journal of Applied Research in Intellectual Disabilities, 19*(2), 179–190. https://doi.org/10.1111/j.1468-3148.2005.00260.x

Taylor, J. L., & Thorne, I. (2005). *Northgate firesetter risk assessment* [Unpublished manual]. Tyne & Wear NHS Foundation Trust.

Taylor, J. L., & Thorne, I. (2013). Pathological firesetting by adults: Assessing and managing risk within a functional analytic framework. In C. Logan & L. Johnstone (Eds.), Managing clinical risk: A guide to effective practice (pp. 142–164). Routledge.

Taylor, J. L., & Thorne, I. (2019). Assessing firesetters with intellectual disabilities. *Journal of Intellectual Disabilities and Offending Behaviour, 10*(4), 102–118. https://doi.org/10.1108/JIDOB-10-2019-0020

Taylor, J. L., Thorne, I., Robertson, A., & Avery, G. (2002). Evaluation of a group intervention for convicted arsonists with mild and borderline intellectual disabilities. *Criminal Behavior and Mental Health, 12*(4), 282–293. https://doi.org/10.1002/cbm.506

Taylor, J. L., Thorne, I., & Slavkin, M. (2004). Treatment of fire-setting behaviour. In W. L. Lindsay, J. L. Taylor & P. Sturmey (Eds.), Offenders with developmental disabilities (pp. 221–240). John Wiley & Sons.

Teasdale, J. D. (1997). The relationship between cognition and emotion: The mind-in-place in mood disorders. In D. M. Clark & C. G. Fairburn (Eds.), Science and practice of cognitive behaviour therapy (pp. 67–93). Oxford University Press.

Teasdale, J. D. (1999). Emotional processing, three modes of mind and the prevention of relapse in depression. *Behaviour Research and Therapy, 37*, S53–S77. https://doi.org/10.1016/S0005-7967(99)00050-9

Teasdale, J. D., & Barnard, P. J. (1993). Affect, cognition and change: Remodelling depressive thought. Lawrence Erlbaum Associates.

Thomson, A., Tiihonen, J., Miettunen, J., Virkkunen, M., & Lindberg, N. (2017). Fire-setting performed in adolescence or early adulthood predicts schizophrenia: A register-based follow-up study of pre-trial offenders. *Nordic Journal of Psychiatry, 71*(2), 96–101. https://doi.org/10.1080/08039488.2016.1233997

Thomson, A., Tiihonen, J., Miettunen, J., Virkkunen, M., & Lindberg, N. (2018). Firesetting and general criminal recidivism among a consecutive sample of Finnish pretrial male firesetters: A register-based follow-up study. *Psychiatry Research, 259*, 377–384. https://doi.org/10.1016/j.psychres.2017.11.008

Tomkins, S. S. (1991). Affect, imagery, consciousness. volume III: The negative affects: Anger and fear. Springer Publishing Co.

Tyler, N., & Gannon, T. A. (2012). Explanations of firesetting in mentally disordered offenders: A review of the literature. *Psychiatry: Interpersonal and Biological Processes, 75*(2), 150–166. https://doi.org/10.1521/psyc.2012.75.2.150

Tyler, N., & Gannon, T. A. (2017). Pathways to firesetting for mentally disordered offenders: A preliminary examination. *International Journal of Offender Therapy and Comparative Criminology, 61*(8), 938–955. https://doi.org/10.1177/0306624X15611127

Tyler, N., & Gannon, T. A. (2021). The classification of deliberate firesetting. *Aggression and Violent Behavior, 59*, 101458. https://doi.org/10.1016/j.avb.2020.101458

Tyler, N., Gannon, T. A., Dickens, G. L., & Lockerbie, L. (2015). Characteristics that predict firesetting in male and female mentally disordered offenders. *Psychology, Crime and Law, 21*(8), 776–797. https://doi.org/10.1080/1068316X.2015.1054382

Tyler, N., Gannon, T. A., Lockerbie, L., King, T., Dickens, G. L., & De Burca, C. (2014). A firesetting offense chain for mentally disordered offenders. *Criminal Justice and Behavior, 41*(4), 512–530. https://doi.org/10.1177/0093854813510911

Tyler, N., Gannon, T. A., Lockerbie, L., & Ó Ciardha, C. (2018). An evaluation of a specialist firesetting treatment programme for male and female mentally disordered offenders (the FIP-MO). *Clinical Psychology & Psychotherapy, 25*(3), 388–400. https://doi.org/10.1002/cpp.2172

Tyler, N., Gannon, T. A., Ó Ciardha, C., Ogloff, J. R. P., & Stadolnik, R. (2019a). Deliberate firesetting: An international public health issue. *The Lancet Public Health, 4*(8), e371–e372. https://doi.org/10.1016/S2468-2667(19)30136-7

Tyler, N., Gannon, T. A., & Sambrooks, K. (2019b). Arson assessment and treatment: The need for an evidence-based approach. *The Lancet Psychiatry, 6*(10), 808–809. https://doi.org/10.1016/S2215-0366(19)30341-4

Tyler, N., Heffernan, R., & Fortune, C. A. (2020). Reorienting locus of control in individuals who have offended through strengths-based interventions: Personal agency and the good lives model. *Frontiers in Psychology, 11*, 2297. https://doi.org/10.3389/fpsyg.2020.553240

van't Veer, A. E., & Giner-Sorolla, R. (2016). Pre-registration in social psychology—A discussion and suggested template. *Journal of Experimental Social Psychology, 67*, 2–12. https://doi.org/10.1016/j.jesp.2016.03.004

Vaughn, M. G., Fu, Q., DeLisi, M., Wright, J. P., Beaver, K. M., Perron, B. E., & Howard, M. O. (2010). Prevalence and correlates of fire-setting in the United States: Results from the National Epidemiological Survey on Alcohol and Related Conditions. *Comprehensive Psychiatry, 51*(3), 217–223. https://doi.org/10.1016/j.comppsych.2009.06.002

Virkkunen, M., DeJong, J., Bartko, J., Goodwin, F. K., & Linnoila, M. (1989). Relationship of psychobiological variables to recidivism in violent offenders and impulsive fire setters. A follow-up study. *Archives of General Psychiatry, 46*(7), 600–603. https://doi.org/10.1001/archpsyc.1989.01810070026003

Virkkunen, M., Nuutila, A., Goodwin, F. K., & Linnoila, M. (1987). Cerebrospinal fluid monoamine metabolite levels in male arsonists. *Archives of General Psychiatry, 44*(3), 241–247. https://doi.org/10.1001/archpsyc.1987.01800150053007

Völlm, B. A., Edworthy, R., Huband, N., Talbot, E., Majid, S., Holley, J., Furtado, V., Weaver, T., McDonald, R., & Duggan, C. (2018). Characteristics and pathways of long-stay patients in high and medium secure settings in England; A secondary publication from a large mixed-methods study. *Frontiers in Psychiatry, 9*, 140. https://doi.org/10.3389/fpsyt.2018.00140

Vreeland, R., & Levin, B. (1980). Psychological aspects of firesetting. In D. Canter (Ed.), Fires and human behaviour (pp. 31–46). Wiley.

Wachi, T., Watanabe, K., Yokota, K., Suzuki, M., Hoshino, M., Sato, A., & Fujita, C. (2007). Offender and crime characteristics of female serial arsonists in Japan. *Journal of Investigative Psychology and Offender Profiling, 4*(1), 29–52. https://doi.org/10.1002/jip.57

Walker, B. L., Beck, K., Walker, A. L., & Shemanski, S. (1992). The short-term effects of a fire safety education program for the elderly. *Fire Technology, 28*(2), 134–162. https://doi.org/10.1007/BF01857941

Walters, G. D. (2016). Animal cruelty and firesetting as behavioral markers of fearlessness and disinhibition: Putting two-thirds of Macdonald's triad to work. *The Journal of Forensic Psychiatry & Psychology, 28*(1), 10–23. https://doi.org/10.1080/14789949.2016.1244856

Walton, J. S. (2019). The evolutionary basis of belonging: Its relevance to denial of offending and labelling those who offend. *Journal of Forensic Practice, 21*(4), 202–211. https://doi.org/10.1108/JFP-04-2019-0014

Ward, T. (2000). Sexual offenders' cognitive distortions as implicit theories. *Aggression and Violent Behavior, 5*(5), 491–507. https://doi.org/10.1016/S1359-1789(98)00036-6

Ward, T. (2010). The Good Lives Model of offender rehabilitation: Basic assumptions, aetiological commitments, and practice implications. In F. McNeill, P. Raynor & C. Trotter (Eds.), Offender supervision: New directions in theory, research and practice (pp. 41–64). Routledge.

Ward, T. (2014). The explanation of sexual offending: From single factor theories to integrative pluralism. *Journal of Sexual Aggression, 20*(2), 130–141. https://doi.org/10.1080/13552600.2013.870242

Ward, T., & Beech, A. (2006). An integrated theory of sexual offending. *Aggression and Violent Behavior, 11*(1), 44–63. https://doi.org/10.1016/j.avb.2005.05.002

Ward, T., & Carter, E. (2019). The classification of offending and crime related problems: A functional perspective. *Psychology, Crime & Law, 25*(6), 542–560. https://doi.org/10.1080/1068316X.2018.1557182

Ward, T., & Hudson, S. M. (1998). The construction and development of theory in the sexual offending area: A metatheoretical framework. *Sexual Abuse: A Journal of Research and Treatment, 10*(1), 47–63. https://doi.org/10.1177/107906329801000106

Ward, T., & Hudson, S. M. (2000). Sexual offenders' implicit planning: A conceptual model. *Sexual Abuse: A Journal of Research and Treatment, 12*(3), 189–202. https://doi.org/10.1023/A:1009534109157

Ward, T., Hudson, S. M., & Marshall, W. L. (1996). Attachment style in sex offenders: A preliminary study. *Journal of Sex Research, 33*(1), 17–26. https://doi.org/10.1080/00224499609551811

Ward, T., & Keenan, T. (1999). Child molesters' implicit theories. *Journal of Interpersonal Violence, 14*(8), 821–838. https://doi.org/10.1177/088626099014008003

Ward, T., Louden, K., Hudson, S. M., & Marshall, W. L. (1995). A descriptive model of the offense chain for child molesters. *Journal of Interpersonal Violence, 10*(4), 452–472. https://doi.org/10.1177/088626095010004005

Ward, T., Mann, R. E., & Gannon, T. A. (2007). The good lives model of offender rehabilitation: Clinical implications. *Aggression and Violent Behavior, 12*(1), 87–107. https://doi.org/10.1016/j.avb.2006.03.004

Ward, T., Polaschek, D. L. L., & Beech, A. R. (2006). Theories of sexual offending. Wiley.

Ward, T., & Stewart, C. A. (2003). The treatment of sex offenders: Risk management and good lives. *Professional Psychology: Research and Practice, 34*(4), 353–360. https://doi.org/10.1037/0735-7028.34.4.353

Ware, J., & Blagden, N. (2020). Men with sexual convictions and denial. *Current Psychiatry Reports, 22*(9), 51. https://doi.org/10.1007/s11920-020-01174-z

Ware, J., Blagden, N., & Harper, C. (2020). Are categorical deniers different? Understanding demographic, personality, and psychological differences between denying and admitting individuals with sexual convictions. *Deviant Behavior, 41*(4), 399–412. https://doi.org/10.1080/01639625.2018.1558944

Ware, J. E., Kosinski, M., Turner-Boweker, D. M., & Gandek, B. (2002). How to score version 2 of the SF-12v2® health survey. QualityMetric Incorporated.

Ware, J., & Marshall, W. L. (2008). Treatment engagement with a sexual offender who denies committing the offense. *Clinical Case Studies, 7*(6), 592–603. https://doi.org/10.1177/1534650108319913

Weerasekera, P. (1996). Multiperspective case formulation: A step towards treatment integration. Krieger Publishing Company.

Williams, D. L. (2005). Understanding the arsonist: From assessment to confession. Lawyers & Judges Publishing Company.

Willis, G. M. (2018). Why call someone by what we don't want them to be? The ethics of labeling in forensic/correctional psychology. *Psychology, Crime & Law, 24*(7), 727–743. https://doi.org/10.1080/1068316X.2017.1421640

Willis, G. M., & Letourneau, E. J. (2018). Promoting accurate and respectful language to describe individuals and groups. *Sexual Abuse, 30*(5), 480–483. https://doi.org/10.1177/1079063218783799

Willis, G. M., Prescott, D. S., & Yates, P. M. (2016). Application of an integrated good lives approach to sexual offending treatment. In D. P. Boer (Ed.), The Wiley handbook on the theories, assessment and treatment of sexual offending (pp. 1355–1368). John Wiley & Sons.

Willis, G. M., Yates, P. M., Gannon, T. A., & Ward, T. (2013). How to integrate the good lives model into treatment programs for sexual offending: An introduction and overview. *Sexual Abuse, 25*(2), 123–142. https://doi.org/10.1177/1079063212452618

Wilpert, J., Van Horn, J., & Eisenberg, M. (2017). Arsonists and violent offenders compared: Two peas in a pod? *International Journal of Offender Therapy and Comparative Criminology, 61*(12), 1354–1368. https://doi.org/10.1177/0306624X15619165

Wolford, M. (1972). Some attitudinal, psychological and sociological characteristics of incarcerated arsonists. *Fire and Arson Investigator, 22*(4), 1–30.

World Health Organization (2011, November 21). *Violence prevention alliance: The public health approach.* Retrieved December 3, 2019, from https://www.who.int/violenceprevention/approach/public_health/e

Wyatt, B., Gannon, T. A., McEwan, T. E., Lockerbie, L., & O'Connor, A. (2019). Mentally disordered firesetters: An examination of risk factors. *Psychiatry, 82*(1), 27–41. https://doi.org/10.1080/00332747.2018.1534520

Index

Note: Page numbers with italic *f* and *t* denote figures and tables respectively.